Principles of or

J. R. MOORE
Emeritus Professor of Oral Surgery in the University of Manchester

G. V. GILLBE
Senior Lecturer in Oral Surgery in the University of Manchester

FOURTH EDITION

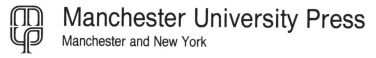

Manchester University Press
Manchester and New York

Distributed exclusively in the USA and Canada by St. Martin's Press

Published by Manchester University Press
Oxford Road, Manchester M13 9PL, UK
and
Room 400, 175 Fifth Avenue, New York
NY 10010, USA

A catalogue record for this book is available from the British Library

Library of Congress cataloging in publication data

Moore, J. R.
    Principles of oral surgery / J. R. Moore, G. V. Gillbe. — 4th ed.
      p.   cm.
    Includes index.
    ISBN 0-7190-3360-8 (pbk.)
    1. Mouth—Surgery.   I. Gillbe, G. V.   II. Title.
    [DNLM: 1. Dentistry, Operative.   2. Surgery, Oral.   WU 600 M822p]
    RK529.M66   1991
    617.5'22059-dc20
    DNLM/DLC
    for Library of Congress   91-19700

ISBN 0 7190 3360 8 paperback

Typeset by Key Graphics, Aldermaston, Berkshire
Printed in Great Britain
by Biddles Ltd, Guildford & King's Lynn

Contents

Foreword to the first edition *Sir Terence Ward*   *page* iv
Preface to the fourth edition   iv

    I   The new patient   1

    II   General patient management   8

    III   Problems related to certain systemic conditions   19

    IV   Emergencies in oral surgery   32

    V   Prescribing for certain common conditions or needs
    in oral surgery *U. J. Moore*   40

    VI   The operating room, instruments and the surgical team   49

    VII   Surgical principles and technique   60

    VIII   Extraction of teeth and roots   75

    IX   Extraction of unerupted teeth   93

    X   Complications of tooth extraction   113

    XI   Preparation of the mouth for dentures *J. W. Frame*   129

    XII   Treatment of surgical infections about the face   144

    XIII   Treatment of cysts of the mouth   160

    XIV   Treatment of fractured jaws *U. J. Moore*   172

    XV   Considerations in the treatment of tumours of the
    mouth *J. G. Cowpe*   205

    XVI   Treatment of surgical conditions of the salivary
    glands *J. G. Cowpe*   220

    XVII   The temporomandibular joint   227

    XVIII   Occlusal and facial disharmony   236

Appendix   246
Index   248
Acknowledgements   252

Foreword to the first edition

There is an increasing need for trained oral surgeons in the world today. An operative field that was a no-man's-land partly controlled by the general surgeon, partly controlled by the dental surgeon, has now come to be the field of a specialised branch of dentistry.

In the past we have had to use books written and published in America, and, fine though these books are, it is refreshing to find a book produced by a British oral surgeon, because in the world today, British oral surgery has undoubtedly the highest general level of training and achievement in the oral surgical field.

Mr J. R. Moore has had considerable practical experience as an oral surgeon in a consultative capacity before devoting his talents to teaching, and he has produced a book of great practical use both to the student or trainee learning oral surgery and also a book of great interest to the established specialist.

I deplore the fragmentation of the dental profession by dividing it into so many specialities, but in the field of oral surgery there are procedures which the dental surgeon would not wish to carry out. Therefore a knowledge of the difficulties and hazards of an oral surgical procedure is essential for the general dental surgeon, who should include this book in his library.

It is with great pleasure that I commend this work of Mr J. R. Moore of University College Hospital to the profession.

T. G. WARD

Preface to the fourth edition

The principles of surgery change little but require modification in the light of newly recognized disease and new treatment modes. Whilst updating the text no attempt has been made to include the more complex procedures performed by maxillofacial surgeons. An introduction to these areas has been included as a basis on which teachers may enlarge as necessary. This remains a book for the undergraduate dental student and a starting point for postgraduates commencing the arduous training for the speciality of oral and maxillofacial surgery.

ı The new patient

It is difficult to overstress the importance of a good history and thorough clinical examination for every patient. On this the diagnosis is made and the treatment plan based. A full, clearly written record of the original consultation is essential to assess progress following treatment. Particularly is this true if a colleague should be called to see the patient in the practitioner's absence. The medicolegal importance of accurate records cannot be overemphasised.

In hospital and specialist practice this procedure can seldom be relaxed, but the student and the busy practitioner may find it irksome to maintain a high standard when faced with a series of apparently straightforward dental conditions. Nevertheless, sufficient time must be allowed for an unhurried consultation at the first visit. This will help to avoid errors of omission, and may contribute much to the success of treatment and to the interest of the practitioner. With experience, only important facts need be noted, the dental surgeon considering and setting aside the irrelevant points. This technique can be used with safety only after a long apprenticeship during which many histories and examinations have been methodically completed and all the information recorded. In this chapter a system for interviewing and examining patients, and recording findings, is briefly suggested.

History

At the first meeting it is important for the clinician to establish a relationship with the patient and to assess his attitude to the clinical situation. He is seated comfortably and addressed by his name and correct title. The general details of age, sex, marital status, occupation and address together with the names of his general medical and dental practitioner are entered in the notes. At this stage it should be possible to determine whether the patient is anxious or relaxed. The history is then recorded under the headings shown in italics.

The patient will seldom tell his story well. Some will be verbose, others reticent, while the sequence is usually in inverse chronological order with the most recent events first. The art of the good history lies in avoiding leading questions, in eliciting all the essentials, in censoring verbosity and in arranging the facts in their true order, so that the written record is short and logical. Allowing the patient initially to give the history and subsequently writing notes in chronological order whilst rechecking the facts verbally, helps the clinician obtain a concise and accurate account of the patient's symptoms.

Patient referred by. The name and professional status of the person referring is noted.

Complains of (C./O.). The patient's chief complaint told *in his own words*. Opinions, professional and otherwise, repeated in an effort to help must be gently set aside and the patient encouraged to describe the symptoms he wants cured, and not his views on the diagnosis.

History of present complaint (H.P.C.). This is an account in *chronological order* of the disease. When and how it first started, the suspected cause, any exciting factors, and the character of the local lesion such as pain, swelling and discharge. This includes remissions and the effects of any treatment received. General symptoms such as fever, malaise and nausea are also noted.

Previous dental history (P.D.H.). This records how regularly the patient attends for dental care and the importance he attaches to his teeth. Any past experience of oral surgery is included especially where difficulty occurred in the administration of anaesthetics, the extraction of teeth and the control of bleeding.

Medical history (M.H.). A summary in chronological order of the patient's past illnesses. Details of prolonged illness, or those requiring hospital admission or current medication are recorded. The surgeon should exert his critical faculty and write down only those conditions that may affect the diagnosis or treatment. The more important of these medical conditions are discussed in Chapter III.

The family history (F.H.). Occasionally this is of importance in oral surgery. Hereditary diseases such as haemophilia and partial anodontia may be relevant in management of the patient.

The social history (S.H.). This includes a brief comment on the patient's occupation and social habits such as exercise, smoking and drinking. The home circumstances are important when surgery is to be performed – that is, whether the patient has far to travel, lives alone or has someone to look after him. These factors may influence the decision to treat him as an in- or out-patient.

Principles of examination

Superficially the dental surgeon's examination may seem very different from that of his medical colleagues, yet the basic principles are the same. It should be made according to a definite system which in time becomes a ritual. In this way errors of omission are avoided.

From the moment the patient enters the surgery he should be carefully observed for signs of physical or of psychological disease which may show in the gait, the carriage, the general manner, or the relationship between parent and child. Too little time is often spent on visual inspection, both intra- and extraorally. Eyes first, then hands, should be the rule, not both together.

In palpation all movements are purposeful and logical, and the touch firm but gentle. The tips of the fingers are used first to locate anatomical landmarks and then to determine the characteristics of the pathological condition. The patient's co-operation is sought so that areas of tenderness may be recognised and the minimum discomfort caused. Wherever possible the normal side is examined simultaneously. Only by such comparison can minor degrees of asymmetry be detected. Swellings situated in the floor of the mouth or in the cheek are felt bimanually with one hand placed in, and one outside, the mouth. Both positive and negative findings are written down as later one may wish to check that at the first visit no abnormality was found in certain structures.

Systematic procedure for examination of the mouth

Extraoral examination

This commences with a general inspection, and palpation of the face including the mandible, maxillary and malar bones, noting the presence of any abnormality such as asymmetry or paralysis of the facial muscles. The eyes, their movements and pupil reactions, are observed together with any difficulty in breathing.

The temporomandibular joints. With the surgeon standing behind the patient, the site of the condyles are identified by palpation whilst the patient opens and closes their mouth. The joints are examined for tenderness and clicking or crepitus on opening and closing. The range of opening and left and right lateral excursion are checked and abnormalities noted. The muscles of mastication are palpated for tenderness.

The maxillary sinuses. In disease these may give rise to swellings, to redness and tenderness over the cheek and canine fossa, to nasal discharge, and to fistulae into the mouth, often through a tooth socket.

The lymph nodes. The operator stands behind the patient, who flexes his head forward to relax his neck muscles. Enlarged submental and submandibular nodes can be felt with the finger tips by placing these below the lower border of the mandible and rolling the nodes outwards. The upper deep cervical group can be found by identifying the anterior border of the sternomastoid muscles and rolling the skin and subcutaneous tissues between fingers and thumb. With practice tenderness, consistency and degrees of mobility will be recognised.

The lips. These are inspected for lesions such as fissuring at the angles of the mouth, or ulceration.

Intraoral examination

The mucous membranes. The cheeks, lips, palate and floor of the mouth are examined for colour, texture and presence of swelling or ulceration. Comparison of both sides by palpation is essential to discover any abnormality.

The tongue.   Movements, both intrinsic and extrinsic, are tested, as limitation is an important clinical sign in inflammation and early neoplasia. The dorsum is best seen by protruding the tongue over a dental napkin with which it can be grasped, drawn forward and, with the aid of a mouth mirror, examined over its length for fissures, ulcers, etc.

The tonsils.   These are seen by depressing the tongue with a spatula and asking the patient to say 'Ah'. A second spatula compresses the anterior pillar of the fauces to evert the tonsil from its bed. Further pressure will expose and open the crypts.

The pharynx.   Again the tongue is depressed, the patient asked to say 'Ah'. In a good light a small warm mirror is passed over the dorsum of the tongue, past the uvula, and rotated to show the naso- and oro-pharynx.

The salivary glands.   The examination of these is described in Chapter XVI.

The periodontal tissues.   The colour and texture of the gingivae are noted, the standard of oral hygiene classified including charting the presence of plaque and calculus. Recession, pocketing, and hyperplasia of the gums is measured, and the mobility of the teeth assessed.

The teeth.   These are charted for caries and fillings with a mirror and probe. Loose teeth, crowns, or fillings are noted as these may have to be removed before a general anaesthetic is administered.

Edentulous ridges.   These are examined for the form of the ridge, retained roots and soft tissue or bony abnormalities. Dentures worn should be inspected *in situ.*

The occlusion.   This is best analysed by taking study models and mounting them on an anatomical articulator. However, the occlusal function of natural teeth, bridges and dentures should be assessed at the same time as the teeth are charted.

Special lesion

This is the examination of the lesion for which the patient has sought treatment. It may have been included in the general examination mentioned above, but frequently there is a swelling, ulcer, fistula or other disease which requires special attention, the details of which are best recorded under one heading easily referred to throughout treatment.

It is important in examining such pathological entities to determine their site, size, shape, colour, the character of their margins and whether they are single or multiple. Tenderness, discharge and lymphatic involvement are also important. Swellings should be palpated to determine whether they are mobile or fixed to the skin or to the underlying tissues. They may be either fluctuant or solid. Solid swellings may be very hard (like bone) or firm (like contracted muscle), soft (like relaxed muscle) or very soft (like fat). Where a collection of fluid is suspected fluctuation is elicited by placing two fingers of one hand on each side of the swelling and pressing centrally with a finger of the other hand. Where the lesion is fluid a thrill will be felt. This must be elicited in two directions at right angles as muscle fluctuates in the longitudinal but not the transverse plane. All pulsatile swellings must be checked to establish whether the pulsation is true or transmitted from an underlying artery.

Special investigation

The history taken, and the examination of the patient having been completed, the surgeon then considers his findings and makes a differential or provisional diagnosis. In this he wishes to establish the disease process and relate it to the tissue involved. It is a useful exercise for the inexperienced to consider in turn the chief pathological categories (Table 1) rejecting those that do not fit the facts ascertained. The tissues in the area may then be reviewed and an attempt made to identify those from which the lesion could arise. In this way a sensible argument may be sustained to support one or more possible or differential diagnoses. To differentiate between these or to confirm a clinical finding special investigations may be necessary. These are not indicated for every patient; indeed, their cost and the delay

Table 1 The surgical sieve. The consideration of possible pathological processes and the tissues involved may be considered as a 'surgical sieve' into one of the holes of which the diagnosis may fit.

Pathological categories		Tissue involved									
		Epithelium	Connective tissue	Fat	Muscle	Bone	Blood vessels	Lymphatics	Nerves	Dental tissues	Salivary gland
Hereditary											
Developmental											
Traumatic											
Inflammatory	(acute)										
	(chronic)										
Cystic											
Neoplastic (benign)											
Neoplastic (malignant)											
Degenerative											
Medical											
Endocrine											

involved in completing them make it necessary to limit their use. Such investigations are an aid to diagnosis and may also be required for treatment planning. It is convenient to divide the more usual procedures into the four main categories shown in Table 2.

Though the dental surgeon may not complete those tests requiring laboratory facilities, yet he must be quite clear about how the necessary specimens are collected and, even more important, understand the clinical significance of the results. These have been dealt with extensively in other works and the method of collection of certain specimens are described later in this text in the appropriate chapter.

Diagnosis

When the special investigations have been completed the surgeon should be able to make a final diagnosis and it is important that this be clearly stated in the notes. Diagnosis is not a matter of intuition but is a 'computer' exercise in which all the information is sorted and analysed in the surgeon's mind. Sometimes it is impossible to reach a decision because of lack of information or knowledge, in which case the surgeon will need to consult textbooks or papers and will be wise to seek the opinion of a colleague.

Treatment planning

Only when the diagnosis is established can a satisfactory treatment plan be made. This should be divided into pre-operative, operative and post-operative care, each of which should be planned in a logical sequence, constantly bearing in mind that the ultimate aim is to cure the patient with the least risk and minimal inconvenience to him.

Further reading

Eastham, R. D. (1987), *Clinical haematology*, 6th edn. John Wright, Bristol.
Fraenkel, G. J. and Ludbrook, J., eds. (1987), *Guide for House Surgeons and Interns in the Surgical Unit*, 8th edn. Heinemann Medical, London.
Macleod, J. and Monroe, J. F., eds. (1986), *Clinical examination*, 7th edn. Churchill Livingstone, Edinburgh.

Table 2 Special investigations commonly used in oral surgery.

Local dental investigations
  A. *Performed in the surgery*

  (i) Percussion of teeth for apical tenderness.
  (ii) Vitality tests on teeth:
    a. Thermal.
    b. Electical.
  (iii) Radiography.
  (iv) Diagnostic injections of local anaesthetic solutions in facial pain.
  (v) Study models for studying the occlusion.
  (vi) Photography as a comparative record.

  B. *Requiring special facilities*

  (i) Bacteriological investigations including sensitivity tests.
  (ii) Aspiration of cystic cavities.
  (iii) Biopsy of tissue.

General investigations

  A. *Performed in the surgery*
  (i) Temperature of body.
  (ii) Pulse rate.
  (iii) Blood pressure.
  (iv) Respiration rate.

  B. *Requiring special facilities*

  (i) Urinalysis.
    Physical examination for colour, specific gravity.
    Chemical, tests for sugar, acetone, albumen, chlorides, blood.
    Microscopic, examination for cells, bacteria, blood.
    Bacteriological culture.
  (ii) Blood investigations:
    Haemoglobin estimation.
    Red cell, white cell and platelet count.
    Bleeding and clotting mechanisms.
    Grouping and cross matching for transfusion.
    Blood chemistry and electrolytes — calcium, inorganic phosphorus, alkaline phosphatase, serum potassium, chloride, albumen, globulin, urea, glucose (see appendix).
    Serology
  (iii) Chest radiographs.
  (iv) Electrocardiograph.
  (v) Tests for allergy.

II   General patient management

The management of surgical patients can be considered under three headings: pre-operative, operative and post-operative; these should form a programme planned to meet the patient's therapeutic need. This chapter is concerned with the pre- and post-operative care, excluding the medically compromised patients, who are the subject of chapter III.

Once the operation has been planned it must be decided whether the patient requires admission to hospital, can be treated on a day-case basis or as an outpatient. The in-patient routine ensures a regular, ordered life with maximum rest. The greater part of the day is taken up by ward rounds and treatment. Smoking is controlled and lights are turned out at 10.30 p.m. Meals, although light and small in quantity, occur frequently at set intervals. This isolation from outside irritations provides an environment which, with the best will in the world, can seldom be achieved at home. Day-stay facilities where the patient is admitted in the morning to return home post-operatively, some hours after recovery, are becoming increasingly popular. The advantages are post-operative supervision by nursing staff during the period when complications related to surgery or anaesthesia may occur, whilst allowing the patient to return home at night. However the home circumstances must be such that the patient can be adequately looked after by relatives. The patient must be within reasonable distance of help post-operatively, should unexpected complications occur. In oral surgery the majority of out-patients are treated using local anaesthesia, sometimes in conjunction with sedation techniques. In-patients usually have endotracheal general anaesthesia of a longer duration than should be administered on a day-stay basis.

The indications for admitting patients to hospital are:

Surgical.   The diagnosis is in doubt and further investigations are needed, the risk of complications such as haemorrhage or fracture of the jaw exists, multiple operations are proposed, or major surgery is being undertaken. In the last respect size alone is no criterion of the importance of the condition.

Medical.   The patient requires collateral treatment by a physician, needs special therapy or skilled nursing care.

Social.   The patient's home conditions are poor, he is living alone, lives far away or he is anxious to be treated as an in-patient.

In patient care demands a wider application of the general principles which underlie the management of surgical patients. It is therefore considered first, though no important difference is implied between the needs of in- and out-patients.

In-patient care

The date of admission to hospital is best arranged at the time of consultation and all waiting lists thereby avoided. Where a waiting list is used it is important to give adequate warning that a bed is available and also to recognise certain surgical priorities such as the following:

Emergency. Conditions requiring instant admission such as acute infections or traumatic injuries.

Urgent. Conditions which can progress to emergencies if treatment is long delayed, for example subacute infections, and neoplasms.

Routine. Those of no urgency who may take their turn in chronological order.

A patient who is fit and only requires routine surgery is normally admitted the day before the operation. Where special preparation is needed such as blood investigation, the fitting of splints or consultation with other specialists, the time of admission must be calculated to allow for these procedures to take place first.

Within a few hours of admission the patient should be visited by the surgeon and findings made at the out-patient examination reviewed and revised if necessary. The pulse, temperature, blood pressure, haemoglobin estimation and urinalysis are recorded. The mouth must be carefully examined and all doubtful cavities in teeth excavated, the caries removed and dressings inserted before surgery. In this way the teeth can be assessed and those beyond conservation extracted under the same anaesthetic. Insecure dressings should be replaced to prevent their being dislodged into a socket or wound. Before a general anaesthetic loose or crowned teeth are noted and the anaesthetist warned. Metal cap splints wherever possible should have been prepared previously as an out-patient and cemented into place twelve hours before they are to be used (Chapter XIV). Where extensive haemorrhage is anticipated blood is taken for grouping and cross matching, and the necessary amount for replacement is ordered. Where grouping is done only as a precautionary measure the serum may be kept for cross matching if required but no blood ordered. The nature of the operation and likely complications should be explained to the patient and permission obtained in writing for both the anaesthetic and the operation. For those under sixteen years of age this permission must be given by the parent or guardian.

It is the role of the dental surgeon not only to carry out the local treatment but also to supervise the day-to-day care.

Relations with the nursing staff

The dental surgeon must understand the routine of the wards and the way his patients are nursed. Though it is essential to make daily visits to assess progress and give treatment, these must be arranged to avoid awkward times when the wards are normally closed. The nursing staff spend much time with the patient and have opportunities to hear complaints and observe minor changes which the surgeon may overlook. Their comments can therefore be of great help and they should be consulted about progress daily.

Consent

Before any procedure is undertaken the patient's consent must be obtained. The proposed operation or investigation should be explained in simple language which can be understood by the lay person. The commoner complications must be mentioned without causing undue distress. Where a general anaesthetic or sedation is proposed the consent should be in writing. For those under sixteen years of age, it must be given by their parent or guardian.

Diet

A knowledge of the principles of nutrition is essential to understand the dietetic problems of the patient, and the following summary is presented with this in mind. The diet can be broadly divided into its fluid and solid content.

Fluid intake and output. The water intake is approximately the sum of the weight expressed in grammes of fluid and of solid food ingested, because solid food when digested and metabolised yields three-fifths its own weight as water. The water intake should be about 2500 ml daily, half of which is taken as drinks.

Water is excreted as exhaled air 400 ml, evaporation including sweat 500–1000 ml, urine 1200 ml, and faeces 200 ml. Water lost by exhalation and evaporation is used for heat regulation and the quantity lost varies widely according to the circumstances. Insufficient fluid intake shows as a decrease in urine output. The absolute daily minimum of urine is the 600 ml required to carry the 50 g of urinary solids excreted daily; below this toxic metabolites are returned to the blood. At this concentration the specific gravity is raised from 1.015 to 1.030. All patients who have difficulty in feeding because of acute trismus or mouth injuries should have a fluid balance chart. This shows on the credit side all fluid taken in twenty-four hours including metabolic water, and on the debit side the urine passed plus an estimate for water lost by evaporation which may be very high in febrile states. For all practical purposes the urine output is a measure of the water balance.

In the adult the daily output should be at least 1000-1500 ml. This simple but accurate criterion is satisfactory unless cardiovascular or renal disease is present, when over-enthusiastic pressing of fluids beyond the power of the kidney to excrete may result in waterlogging of the tissues. Fluids may be administered by several routes, of which only the oral and intravenous are much used. The safest, most convenient and effective way of giving fluids is by mouth and should be preferred to all others. Up to three litres of water, flavoured attractively, can be taken each day. Where the intraoral route cannot be used fluids may be given intravenously.

Solid food. A balanced diet includes carbohydrates, fats, proteins, vitamins and mineral salts.

Fats, the highest calorie provider, are not easily digested by the sick and their intake may have to be markedly reduced. They are, however, important as a vehicle for the fat-soluble vitamins A, D, E and K. In starvation the body's fat reserves may be mobilised, but a certain minimum daily quantity of carbohydrate is needed for their physiological use and to prevent ketosis. Only 100 g of glycogen is stored in the liver, which is less than a one-day requirement. Protein is essential for the repair of tissues, and for maintaining the circulation. A deficiency may occur after extensive haemorrhage or burns and may increase the susceptibility to shock, impede the healing of wounds, impair circulatory efficiency, and lower resistance to infection. Patients in bed undergo protein wastage which is best prevented by a high carbohydrate and protein diet. Vitamins and mineral salts are essential and are supplied therapeutically, if deficient. Complan, a whole food, contains fat 16 g, carbohydrate 44 g, and protein 31 g, per 100 g and includes all necessary minerals and vitamins.

Food must be attractively prepared, and even if sieved or in fluid form it should not lose its identity. Each meal should bear some resemblance to its usual form; most foods can be easily liquidised and baby foods though expensive are useful in this respect.

Special dietary requirements must be discussed with the dietitian and the ward sister. The total calories, the amount of water, protein and vitamins, together with proprietary preparations and the number and the kind of supplementary feeds, must be specified. The rule 'a little and often' will help to avoid indigestion, and to ensure an adequate intake particularly when the jaws are wired together. Thus supplementary feeds should be given so that the daily routine includes early morning tea, breakfast, 'elevenses', lunch, tea, dinner, supper and nightcap. A suitable supplementary feed can be made up with Complan, 3 g dissolved in 0.5 l of milk, suitably flavoured.

Certain patients may have to be fed through a nasogastric (Ryle's) tube. This is a small-bore plastic tube passed through the nose so that about 5 cm lies in the stomach. The normal length of tube from the nose is 50 cm; any excess interferes with gastric peristalsis and may cause anorexia and nausea. Its presence in the stomach is confirmed by aspirating gastric contents up the tube before feeding is started. Feeding may be continued in this way indefinitely if, every two or three days, the tube is brought out, cleaned and replaced through the other nostril. Before use, air present in the stomach is aspirated; the liquid feed is then given with a bulb syringe. Before disconnecting the syringe the nasogastric tube must be clamped off. All patients on special diets should be weighed weekly as a check on their progress.

Pre-operative diet. Patients for operation under local anaesthesia may take their normal meals. If the patient has missed a meal he should be given a glucose drink before the injection is given. Where a general anaesthetic is to be administered a light meal, chiefly of protein and carbohydrate, is advised the night before. On the day of operation those on the morning list are starved, but those for the afternoon list may be given a small breakfast of tea and toast. No food or drink must be taken for at least six hours before operation.

Post-operative diet. Each patient must be considered individually, but feeding should be started as soon as possible to avoid nausea. Many can manage the ordinary fare provided, but others, because of tenderness or trismus, require specially prepared food. Where necessary the patient before discharge home should receive a diet sheet with a list of suitable recipes.

Excretion

Micturition. This reflex act occurs when the pressure in the bladder rises sufficiently to cause the sphincter to relax and the detrusor muscle to contract. The ability to delay micturition is the inhibition of the normal reflex response to distension. In patients with head injuries the apparently insane desire to get out of bed is often for the purpose of emptying the bladder or bowel, as the wish to go to the right place is strongly imbued and may persist despite gross craniocerebral disturbance. Retention can be organic, as in men suffering from prostatic enlargement, or a functional disorder. It may occur after general anaesthesia but should cause no undue anxiety up to twenty-four hours unless the bladder becomes distended or symptoms of overflow occur, Micturition can be encouraged by getting the patient up but if this fails the advice of a genitourinary surgeon should be obtained.

Sweat. This contains 0.5 per cent of solids, chiefly sodium chloride. In fever or in hot weather sweating may be greatly increased and as much as 10 g of sodium chloride can be lost in an hour, which must be replaced in the diet.

Defaecation. The bowels should be regularly opened and the fact noted but too much attention can be paid to irregularity. In constipation one must first decide whether the cause is organic or functional. Organic is due to partial obstruction of the lumen, often by a tumour. Functional may be due to defective movements of the colonic musculature, or a deficiency in bulk of faeces due to feeding with fluid diets. It may arise in hospital as a result of a sudden change in routine and of diet.

It is treated either by feeding fruit, vegetables and wholemeal cereals or by giving laxatives. It is stressed that wherever there is doubt as to the cause a general surgeon's opinion should be sought.

Sleep

Sleep is distinguished from other unconscious states by the ease with which the sleeper may be roused. Disturbed sleep may be due to pain, to external stimuli, to worry or to change of habit. It is important to recognise the cause before considering treatment. Where this is pain, hypnotics must not be given until its source has been investigated, removed if possible, or analgesics prescribed. If these are effective the patient should sleep naturally. External stimuli should be reduced by keeping the wards dark at night, and by providing side wards for night admissions and for the noisy or restless patients. Worry or change of habit, particularly dozing by day, can lead to insomnia in the convalescent or fit adult. Hypnotic drugs may be prescribed, but only if really necessary for they are habit-forming.

Hygiene

General and oral hygiene is the responsibility of the ward sister, but mouth hygiene is supervised by the dental surgeon. On admission the patient should be given a dental prophylaxis and instructed in oral hygiene.

In the badly injured, the elderly and in those recently operated upon, a modified technique is necessary either to avoid causing pain or because they need assistance. No cleansing of the mouth is advised for the first twenty-four hours after operation and may indeed do harm by starting haemorrhage. Thereafter, mucous membranes and teeth may be cleansed with a soft tooth-brush or cotton wool swabs attached to orange sticks, and the mouth irrigated with 0.2 per cent aqueous chlorhexidine after every meal. Intraoral sutures also require care as they tend to trap food over the wound. Clinging debris should be removed by swabbing with cotton wool each day. A hypertonic saline mouth bath may be used as hot as the individual can bear without scalding and allowed to lie over the wound until cool, but unlike the mouth-washes used pre-operatively, no violent flushing is advised. Mouth-brushing is started on normal teeth and gingivae as soon as possible and the patient encouraged at an early stage to carry out his own oral hygiene. This not only occupies his time usefully, but the techniques may be supervised before discharge, ensuring satisfactory home care.

Splints. Metal cap splints may be cleaned with a toothbrush and paste, and Gunning's splints with a mouthbrush or cotton wool swabs using chlorhexidine mouthwash.

In cleft palate and buccal inlay surgery where gutta-percha moulds are used to hold skin grafts in position the mouth is cleansed using only the blandest mouthwashes. After the first ten days (by which time the graft should have taken) a syringe may be introduced between the graft and the mould to clean the dead space gently but thoroughly.

Premedication and sedation. See Chapter V

Post-operative care

On arriving in the recovery room after an operation the patient is immediately put into a warm bed and laid on his side with a pillow behind his shoulders in the position of sleep in such a way that drainage may take place from his mouth. His arms are kept folded over his chest. Under no circumstances should the arms be elevated above his head for fear of damage to the brachial plexus.

During the uneasy period before complete consciousness is regained, and especially where the jaws are wired together, a nurse must sit with the patient to watch the airway, suck out the mouth and oropharynx, ensure that he does himself no injury by pulling at sutures or splints or, as can happen, fall out of bed. She also watches for vomiting, haemorrhage, records the pulse, blood pressure, respirations, and level of consciousness.

Post-operative medication

Analgesics should be given to reduce post-operative pain. Hypnotics should not be prescribed for semi-conscious patients where the jaws are wired together (see Chapter V).

Post-operative complications

These can include fever, vomiting, conjunctivitis, sore throat, pharyngitis and pulmonary conditions.

Fever. Raised temperature is a natural reaction to infection but a slight fever is common for two to three days after an operation where a haematoma or necrotic material is present. A large haematoma may keep the temperature up for a week. After a general anaesthetic the dental surgeon must consider a chest complication as a cause of fever. More rarely a temporary upset of heat regulation does occur after an anaesthetic or a head injury.

The primary treatment must be that of the underlying cause whether local or general. The symptomatic treatment includes confinement to bed, liberal administration of fluids and a high carbohydrate diet which has been found to prevent the breakdown of body proteins. At temperatures of 39.4 °C and over, the body may be sponged down with tepid water at 27 °C which cools the patient and refreshes him.

Vomiting. This does occur following operation, usually due to the anaesthetic or swallowed blood, though the nervous disposition of the patient is a factor Persistent vomiting for more than eight hours is part of a vicious circle characterised by an upset of the acid base equilibrium, in which the alkali reserve is reduced with increased urinary acidity and ketonuria. For the treatment of this the anaesthetist should be consulted. It can however often be avoided by energetic treatment earlier. This consists of giving milk or alkaline drinks with glucose, which should be sipped very slowly but frequently. An antiemetic may be prescribed (Chapter V).

Conjunctivitis. Conjunctivitis can be caused by anaesthetic vapours, blood, antiseptics or towels entering the eye, or by the eye being open and drying up during the operation. This can be prevented by keeping the eyes closed with eyepads, but should contamination occur the eye can be gently irrigated with normal saline. Chloramphenicol eye-drops will afford relief.

Sore throat or pharyngitis. This is usually caused by trauma from the endotracheal tube, excoriation from a dry pack or desiccation following use of atropine. It may be treated with gargles and inhalations (Chapter V).

Pulmonary complications. Routine post-operative breathing exercises will reduce the incidence of pulmonary complications but the dental surgeon must bear in mind that they may occur. These may range from a minor inflammation of the trachea or bronchi to pulmonary collapse or post-operative pneumonia. Where they are suspected a chest radiograph should be taken and the anaesthetist immediately informed. Their general management will include the use of antibiotics, physiotherapy, humidified oxygen, sedatives and mucolytic drugs. Frequent hot drinks help to relieve spasm and loosen secretions.

Progress

The patient should be visited daily by the surgeon, who should first ask the patient how he feels and about his day-to-day care, diet and oral hygiene. This is followed by a careful examination of the operation site, a check of the temperature chart, drug sheet, etc., and questions to the nursing staff where necessary. The response to treatment is assessed and should be recorded in the notes, together with any changes to be made in the treatment. Before discharge the patient's final condition should be summarised. The importance of these records cannot be overstressed as it is difficult to compare progress over a long period without them.

Discharge

When the patient is fit for discharge home the patient or the relatives must be informed of the regime and treatment to be followed and when to attend for review. Sick benefit notes must be completed and adequate transport, if necessary, arranged both to the patient's home and for his return for review.

The patient's doctor and dental surgeon should receive notification that the patient is being discharged, including an outline of the operative procedures and condition on discharge. In this way, if called in an emergency, they are informed of all that has gone before, and they are able to prescribe for any drugs or dressings required at home.

Intensive care

Not all patients will follow the above routine; some will be admitted shocked, unconscious or both. Some will require special management after operation and the condition of others may deteriorate whilst they are on the ward. In the modern hospital the critically ill patients are treated in an intensive care unit by specialised staff.

The management of respiration may require intubation or tracheostomy and, on occasion, the use of a mechanical ventilator. Such care is entirely within the realm of a specialist, usually an anaesthetist. Fluids and feeding for these patients is often given intravenously. All prolonged intravenous infusion requires the most careful continual monitoring as it is all too easy to upset the delicately balanced homeostasis.

Intravenous fluids. The solution must be sterile and should be contained in a bottle with a filter to which a polythene tube is attached. All air should be removed from the tube by running the fluid through it with the stop clamp open and alternately raising and lowering the bottle. A suitable vein, not too superficial nor near a joint, is chosen and a tourniquet is placed above the selected point. The needle of the giving set is introduced into the vein and the tourniquet removed, with blood flowing from the needle and fluid from the polythene tube of the bottle the two are connected together. The needle should be firmly strapped into place and the arm fixed to a board to avoid movement. The flow is usually adjusted to 50 drops a minute, the equivalent of 3000 ml in twenty four hours. The reservoir must *not* run dry or an air embolism may occur.

The fluids that may be given in this way are whole blood, plasma and saline, dextrose or fat solutions. The decision as to which fluid to use will depend on the clinical needs of the patient. Blood may be given as a replacement following loss from trauma or surgery and saline or dextrose solutions during long operations and the immediate recovery period; where the use of intravenous fluids goes beyond this short term, monitoring is performed using a central venous pressure line and by taking blood samples and estimating blood sugar and electrolytes. Where feeding using fat solutions is necessary urinary urea estimation and body weight will indicate the nitrogen to be replaced and the calories required.

Out-patient care

All the principles of management of in-patient care, particularly those relating to diet, hygiene and progress, are applicable with modification to out-patients. The salient points with regard to outpatients are summarised here.

Day cases. Where outpatients are having minor operations under endotracheal anaesthesia they may be operated during the morning but kept in a suitably equipped recovery room or ward under adequate professional and nursing supervision. As it is usual for these patients to stay on the premises all day and be discharged home in the evening they are known as 'day cases' though otherwise their general care is the same as that of other out-patients. However they must be examined by the anaesthetist before they are accepted for out-patient anaesthesia. Suitable transport must be available and they will require rest and care on their return home. It is wise before planning such a procedure to involve the general medical practitioner, particularly for assurance that the patient's home circumstances are equal to the situation and that the medical practitioner is prepared to attend the patient should the family call him for advice or assistance in the immediate post-operative period.

Finally both the anaesthetist and the surgeon should be able and experienced in their fields so that the patient is not exposed to risk due to lack of skill or judgement.

Pre-operative instructions for out-patients. The nature of the operation must be explained and the patient's permission obtained in writing for both general anaesthetic and surgery. Out-patients should be told to come accompanied and whether it will be safe to take alcohol, drive a car or bicycle, or operate machinery (including housewives' cooking). Instructions should be given about diet before a local anaesthetic – something light and easily digested. Where a general anaesthetic is to be administered they are instructed to come accompanied, to wear no restrictive clothing and to fast from food or drink for at least six hours before operation; in this respect children require particular supervision. Patients having sedation should be given similar instructions to those having a general anaesthetic. Of particular importance is the advice that the patient must not drive a motor vehicle or operate machinery until the following day. Before entering the surgery they are asked to remove their dentures, contact lenses and earrings, and to empty bowel and bladder.

Pre-operative dental treatment. Pre-operative prophylaxis and instruction in oral hygiene is given to those about to undergo a dental operation. Many patients fail to appreciate the importance of this measure, All doubtful teeth should be assessed and insecure dressings replaced so that those beyond conservation can be extracted under the same anaesthetic. Before a general anaesthetic very loose teeth should be noted and the anaesthetist warned.

Pre- and post-medication. This is discussed in Chapter V.

Post-operative care. Before dismissing the patient, a reasonable time should be allowed for recovery. This applies equally to those treated under local or general anaesthesia, and particularly to day intubation patients.

Adequate instructions should be given for home treatment. If possible these should be stated in the presence of a relative or written, as the patient may not be sufficiently alert after the surgical ordeal to remember details. These should include diet, oral hygiene, analgesics and the rest period required before return to work. The date and time of the next appointment must also be clearly stated, together with the action to be taken should a post-operative emergency, such as haemorrhage, arise (Table 3).

Table 3 Specimen of post-operative instructions to patient

To prevent bleeding
   AVOID mouthwashing for twenty-four hours
      hot drinks, hot food and alcohol
      exercise or effort

If bleeding occurs
   Apply pressure by biting on to a clean rolled handkerchief
   Rest sitting in an upright position
   If bleeding is not controlled by these measures contact us by telephone by day 123-4567,
      by night 123-8901

If in pain
   Take two paracetamol tablets.
   If pain is persistent or severe contact the dental surgery

After 24 hours
   Mix one teaspoonful of salt in a tumbler of hot water
   Take a mouthful and tilt head so that the water lies over the extraction site.
   Hold water over area, spit it out and repeat until the tumbler is empty

Operation . . . .
Anaesthetic. . . . .

The operator *must be easily available* to the patient to deal with any surgical complications which may arise. Where a general anaesthetic has been given, the general medical practitioner should be informed.

Follow-up

It is the duty of the surgeon to assume responsibility for the patient's after-care until all possibility of post-operative complications is past. Though often tedious, long-term follow-up should be carried out personally, as through it much may be learned which will benefit both the surgeon and his patients. Before final discharge, the surgeon should refer back through the notes and establish that not only have the operations been successful, but that the patient has been relieved of his original complaint and that any subsequent complications incurred during treatment have been cured.

Further reading

Ferguson, D. B. (1988), *Physiology for Dental Students*. John Wright, Bristol.
Porte, J. C. and Green, D. W. (1986), *A New Short Textbook of Anaesthetics, Intensive Care and Pain Relief*. Hodder & Stoughton, London.
Poswillo, D., Babajews, A., Bailey, M. and Foster, M. E. (1986), *Dental, Oral and Maxillofacial Surgery: A Guide to Hospital Practice*. Heinemann Medical, London.

III Problems related to certain systemic conditions

The dental surgeon is often asked to undertake oral surgery for patients suffering from systemic diseases or undergoing treatment with drugs, either of which may complicate the operation, including the choice and administration of an anaesthetic. Where surgical procedures cause an exacerbation of the medical condition it is the physician who will treat it, not the dental surgeon. Nothing is more calculated to annoy a general medical practitioner than to be called unexpectedly to advise one of his chronically ill patients who has undergone a surgical operation about which he has not been informed.

A full medical history is therefore essential and should be rechecked periodically if the patient attends for a prolonged period. Whenever a patient is under treatment by a physician the latter must be informed of the proposed operation and his co-operation sought with the pre- and post-operative care, particularly with regard to the special precautions necessary for the disease. No alteration should be made to the drug regime without such prior consultation. Advances in drug therapy occur rapidly in the modern world, and where a patient is on medication with which the dental surgeon is not familiar reference should be made to the British National Formulary.

The more important conditions commonly met in practice will now be discussed.

Physiological conditions

Menstruation

This is not a contraindication to surgery except that patients are often depressed physically and mentally, and this time is best avoided. It has been stated that haemorrhage after extractions is prolonged during this period, but no increase in the bleeding or clotting time of clinical significance has been demonstrated.

Pregnancy

In general, women in pregnancy undergo operations and anaesthesia well, if not better than at other times. The physical or psychological trauma of extraction does not endanger the foetus though it may be blamed for so doing. A local anaesthetic with adrenalin is satisfactory as the hormonal mechanism shields the uterus from smooth muscle activators. In general anaesthesia the greatest danger to the foetus is anoxia, which, even if slight, may have serious, even fatal, results at any time. This is most likely to occur later in pregnancy, especially in the last three months, because the size of the uterus reduces the vital capacity of the mother's lungs, and because the oxygen supply to the human foetus in a normal pregnancy falls slowly to the thirty sixth week and rapidly thereafter.

General anaesthesia in the dental chair should be avoided late in pregnancy as it is more likely to cause complications, owing to the sitting position of the patient, which tends to compress the abdominal contents and so restrict respiratory movement. Further, a nitrous oxide and oxygen anaesthetic is more likely to cause anoxia. However, in a normal pregnancy a short anaesthetic can be given if adequate oxygenation is maintained throughout.

The optimum time for operation is the fourth and fifth months of pregnancy because at that time the danger to the foetus is least. Most frequently abortions occur in the first three months so this period should be avoided, as should the last month in view of the possibility of precipitating premature labour. Certain patients give a history of habitual abortion at other times, and for these surgery should not be undertaken at that particular time.

Many expectant mothers suffer from anaemia, and as this may increase the danger of anoxia to the foetus, the haemoglobin level should be ascertained before any operation is commenced.

Endocrine diseases

Hyperthyroidism

In hyperthyroidism either oral surgery or the injection of local anaesthetic containing adrenalin may precipitate a thyroid crisis. For these reasons surgery must be delayed until the physician is satisfied that the patient is adequately prepared. A general anaesthetic may be preferable to local anaesthesia as it is less upsetting psychologically.

Adrenal corticosteriods

The adrenal cortex produces hormones which are of importance to the surgeon since amongst their functions they affect the balance of electrolytes, depress the inflammatory response and play a large part in the body's reaction to stress. Their secretion is stimulated by the adrenocorticotrophic hormone (ACTH), produced by the anterior lobe of the pituitary. When the amount of adrenocortical hormone in the circulation reaches the necessary level, production of ACTH is inhibited.

Corticosteriods or their synthetic equivalents are used in medicine for replacement therapy of insufficiency which may be chronic primary as in Addison's disease, or chronic secondary as in hypopituitarism. They are also used in the treatment of a wide variety of medical conditions including asthma and the collagen diseases. Where the blood level of the adrenocortical steriods is kept high for therapeutic purposes the adrenal cortex atrophies and causes an iatrogenic insufficiency. Any sudden demand under conditions of stress cannot be met, with the result that an acute adrenal insufficiency (Addisonian crisis) may occur with all the signs and symptoms of shock. Depression of function may continue for years after their therapeutic use has stopped and those who require a general anaesthetic or surgery must have adequate premedication with steriods as advised by their physician. During the operation hydrocortisone sodium succinate must be available. Should a crisis supervene 100 mg should be injected at once intravenously or intramuscularly and an intravenous transfusion started of 0.9 per cent (154 m.mols/l) saline, containing a second 100 mg of the hydrocortisone sodium succinate.

Metabolic disorders

Diabetes

Diabetes mellitus is a disease characterised by a rise in blood sugar, excretion of sugar and acetone in the urine, and an increased susceptibility to infection. Emotional stress or infection may increase the severity of the disease. Broadly the patients may be considered in two groups. The elderly group, often overweight, who develop diabetes later in life. They are non-insulin-dependent diabetics and are treated where necessary with oral hypoglycaemic agents. The second group are insulin-dependent diabetics. Their management is more complex and requires the administration of insulin. In uncontrolled diabetes, hyperglycaemic coma may occur, but this is of slow onset and the patient is so obviously ill beforehand that it is unlikely to present as an emergency in the dental surgery.

However, hypoglycaemia (insulin shock) can occur with alarming suddenness in patients on insulin who have taken insufficient carbohydrate. Weakness, hunger, pallor, a rapid pulse and profuse sweating herald its onset, which if severe is followed by confusion and loss of consciousness. Treatment is to give sugar by mouth or 1 mg glucagon intramuscularly. The patient must be observed to ensure that treatment is adequate.

Where a diabetic is to have an operation under local anaesthesia he should take his normal diet and insulin at the usual time and the operation should be commenced about one hour after. It is not necessary to use adrenalin-free local anaesthetic solutions, but the operation must not be unduly prolonged, nor must meals or snacks on the patient's schedule be missed.

Those on insulin who have an acute infection or need a general anaesthetic should undoubtedly be admitted to hospital, where the advice of a physician may be sought. When a general anaesthetic is to be given the physician will manage the case according to the following broad principles. Those on long-acting insulin are changed to the soluble form and rebalanced. All but the most severe diabetics will then receive their normal insulin and carbohydrate till midnight on the day before operation. Next morning they should be operated first and are given only a saline infusion during the operation, after which a blood sugar estimation is immediately performed before administering the necessary insulin and glucose by infusion. Post-operatively, careful monitoring of the patient and urine testing is continued till the normal balance is resumed.

For severe diabetics or where a long operation is involved more complicated management may be required.

The surgeon must take measures to control infection at the site of operation by careful oral prophylaxis, dentures are provided as quickly as possible so that the patient can resume his normal diet.

Angioedema

Angioedema is a disease in which there is widespread oedema due to increased vascular permeability as a result of an allergic reaction. Two forms exist; one is hereditary and is an apparently exaggerated response to minor trauma and is characteristically shared by other members of the family. Patients are treated with steroids and, as minor operations may cause a severe response, premedication with antihistamines is indicated.

The non-hereditary variety is a kind of urticaria in which there is an allergic response not only to food and drugs, but also to emotional situations. Trauma seldom produces serious complications but the use of allergenic substances may do so. Should an acute reaction occur it should be treated as for anaphylactic shock described in Chapter IV.

Cardiovascular disorders

There are many heart conditions but the dental surgeon is concerned firstly with those which affect the efficiency of the heart as a pump, and secondly those where the valvular endocardium is damaged and susceptible to infection.

Cardiac failure

The symptoms of heart failure are a reduced exercise tolerance, cyanosis, dyspnoea and oedema of the lower extremities. The patient in early failure may not present with these but leads an apparently normal life. Though he has a loss of cardiac reserve this is apparent only when the extra demands made by physical exercise or hypoxia cannot be met.

Failure of the heart to act as an efficient pump occurs in many diseases including congenital heart disease, cardiac arrhythmias, hyperthyroidism, coronary heart disease, hypertension and rheumatic carditis. Patients suffering from these should not be operated upon without a physician's advice as those in failure may be greatly improved by admission to hospital for bed rest and medical treatment. The anaesthetic of choice for these patients is a local anaesthetic. Premedication with a suitable anxiolytic drug should be considered if the patient is unduly concerned about the proposed operation.

Coronary artery disease

Disease of the coronary vessels, because it causes ischaemia of the heart muscle, affects the efficiency of the heart as a pump. Where partial occlusion of the vessels is present severe pain of short duration, called angina of effort, occurs during physical or emotional stress because the demand for blood by the myocardium outstrips the possible supply. Treatment includes the use of vasodilators when pain is experienced. Details of the frequency of need for these tablets will give an indication of the severity of the disease. Where use of the drug is frequent, or increasing in frequency, advice should be sought from the patient's physician. Complete occlusion of a coronary artery is known as a coronary thrombosis, when the patient has acute pain of long duration and is very ill or may die suddenly.

Patients suffering from coronary disease should be treated in conjunction with a physician and should be admitted when a general anaesthetic is required. Some may be on treatment with anticoagulants and obviously require special preparation (see page 27). Those operated under local anaesthesia should be adequately premedicated to allay anxiety, and kept in the supine position to reduce strain on the heart. The use of a local anaethetic solution containing octapressin is indicated. Those using glyceryl trinitrate tablets should be asked to take one before the operation starts – the vasodilator effect lasts about half an hour.

Should an anginal attack occur, the patient is laid down and a 0.5 mg tablet of glyceryl trinitrate is placed under the tongue or a 5 mg sorbide nitrate tablet can be chewed. Oxygen is administered at 6 litres/minute. Where the severity of the attack is marked by cyanosis, cold sweat and dyspnoea suggesting a coronary thrombosis the patient is laid down, given oxygen, and morphine sulphate 20 mg subcutaneously to ease the pain. The patient should be referred to hospital and not sent directly home.

Infective endocarditis

The endocardium of the heart valves may be damaged, as happens in certain congenital heart diseases, in rheumatic fever and Huntington's chorea or following cardiac surgery. The dental surgeon must realise that in these cases the heart may function completely satisfactorily as a pump, yet it may still be susceptible to infection from a bacteraemia at any time during the patient's life. Amongst infecting organisms *Streptococcus viridans* has repeatedly been shown to be released into the blood stream during tooth extraction or oral prophylaxis.

Protection must be afforded to all those with a history of congenital heart disease, rheumatic fever, chorea, or who have had cardiac surgery by an antibiotic umbrella as advised by the physician concerned. Typically this may be one dose of 3 g amoxycillin orally one hour pre-operatively. For those who are allergic to penicillin oral erythromycin stearate is given, one dose of 1.5 g one hour pre-operatively and 500 mg six hours later. For those having a general anaesthetic, 1 mg amoxycillin may be given by intramuscular injection followed by 500 mg orally six hours later. Where there is a history of an episode of endocarditis or the patient has prosthetic replacement of a heart valve, 1 g amoxycillin and 1.5 mg/kg gentamycin are given intramuscularly to be followed by 500 mg oral amoxycillin six hours later. For this latter group who are allergic to penicillin, intravenous vancomycin and gentamycin are given.

Hypertension

Hypertensive patients can trouble the dental surgeon in two ways. First, the raised blood pressure may be a cause of post-operative bleeding as it may prevent the normal vascular and platelet mechanism from arresting haemorrhage effectively. Second, those under treatment with anti-hypertensive drugs can be more susceptible to the hypotensive effects of general anaesthetics, making it necessary to inform the anaesthetist of their use.

Prosthetic joints and valves

Patients suffering from cardiac lesions or congenital hydrocephalus may have artificial valves inserted. These are at risk of infection when a bacteraemia occurs. There is also some evidence that replacement of the head of the femur or other similar joint prostheses are also susceptible. Such patients should be protected by prophylactic antibiotics when extractions are performed.

Disorders of the blood

Anaemia

The oral surgeon must satisfy himself that the patient is not clinically anaemic before operation, and where doubt exists a haemoglobin estimation and blood film examination must be performed. It should always be remembered that there are several different forms of anaemia and that it can be symptomatic of serious disease such as leukaemia, which requires investigation by a haematologist. In severe anaemia operation is delayed until it has responded to treatment or in an emergency a blood transfusion has been arranged.

Sickle cell anaemia

This haemoglobinopathy is a hereditary disease found in individuals of African, Asian and Mediterranean origin. The abnormal haemoglobin (HbS) in lowered oxygen tension (such as may occur during a general anaesthetic) results in the red corpuscle becoming sickle-shaped, leading to an increased blood viscosity and capillary thrombosis. It can present either as true sickle cell anaemia or as sickle cell trait in which there is a variable proportion of affected haemoglobin, the remainder being normal.

All patients who may have inherited the disease and require a general anaesthetic should be tested for sickling (sickledex test). Positive patients require further investigation by a haematologist to differentiate those with the trait from those with sickle cell anaemia. Both groups are more safely treated under local anaesthesia, but where a general anaesthetic is necessary the patient should be referred to hospital for a specialist anaesthetic opinion.

Thalassaemias

These inherited diseases are seen in Mediterranean races in whom foetal haemoglobin continues to be produced after birth. The patients suffer from haemolytic anaemia and should be treated in hospital.

Leukaemias

All forms of leukaemia are a contraindication to any form of oral surgery without full investigation and advice from a haematologist, owing to the difficulty of controlling post-operative bleeding and infection. In such cases a conservative approach to dental care should be adopted until the leukaemia is in remission or the patient is free of the disease.

Haemorrhagic diseases

The natural arrest of haemorrhage is brought about in three ways, first by the contraction of the vessel walls, second by plugging of small deficiencies by platelets, and third by the clotting of the blood. Clinically, patients with haemorrhagic disease can be divided into those where bleeding is profuse at operation and continues, these have a prolonged bleeding time but clotting may be normal. Second, those where bleeding usually stops for a short period after operation but persistent haemorrhage occurs later owing to failure of the blood to clot; these may have a normal bleeding time, but an abnormality of coagulation.

Prolonged bleeding time

This is found where vascular damage prevents arrest by the contraction of the walls of cut vessels or in platelet abnormalities in which there is ineffective plugging of small deficiencies.

Disorders of blood vessels

These occur in anaphylactoid (allergic) purpura of Henoch and Schonlein, in symptomatic purpura as in scurvy, in severe infections such as scarlet fever, following the use of certain drugs, and in hereditary haemorrhagic telangiectasia.

Platelet abnormalities

These are of two kinds: thrombocytopenic purpuras where there is a low platelet count which may be primary as in idiopathic purpura or secondary to drugs or other blood diseases such as leukaemia; and thrombocythaemic purpura in which the platelet count is greatly raised, the condition being related to polycythaemia.

Abnormal coagulation

Table 4 shows the clotting mechanism. There are several theories, of which the waterfall concept is one. The extrinsic mechanism is activated by damaged tissue, whereas the intrinsic is tivated by contact of blood with a surface other than blood cells or endothelium.

Coagulation defects are rare and may arise from a deficiency of any of the factors concerned in the mechanism. The most common disease due to insufficiency of Factor VIII is haemophilia A, a sex-linked disease present in males, but female carriers have lowered levels of Factor VIII which may require correction for surgery. Deficiency of Factor IX causes haemophilia B (Christmas disease), seen in males.

Clotting failure may also occur for want of prothrombin, which is formed in the liver, and vitamin K is necessary for its synthesis.

Table 4 Blood clotting process. Note the extrinsic pathway involves few steps and occurs rapidly.

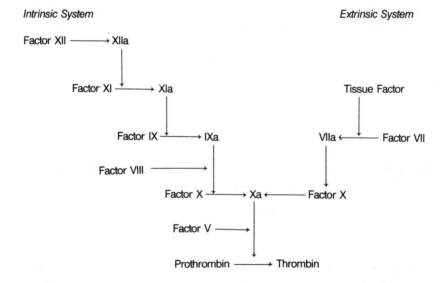

a indicates activated factor.

Fibrinolysis. Normal circulating blood contains plasminogen which is the precursor of plasmin, a proteolytic enzyme which breaks down fibrin and fibrinogen and thereby causes the destruction of clots. Though playing a physiological role in the organisation of clots, excessive fibrinolysis can occur in a wide variety of conditions as in sepsis, acute haemorrhage or after major surgery, thus delaying haemostasis.

Von Willebrand's disease. Von Willibrand's factor (VWF) prolongs the life of F VIII in the circulation and stabilises platelet plugs. Deficiency affects the level of F VIII and platelet function. The disease is seen in males and females.

Anticoagulant therapy. Certain patients will be found who are being treated with anticoagulant drugs following thrombosis or cardiac surgery. Two types of anticoagulant are in use, the rapid and short-acting heparin group which are antithrombins and thereby prevent the conversion of fibrinogen to fibrin, and the longer-acting oral group (their effect may last for days), which reduce the amount of circulating prothrombin by preventing its formation in the liver. Patients on anticoagulant therapy should never be taken off these drugs except on a physician's advice. Before surgery is performed the prothrombin level must be checked and where this is in the therapeutic range within which spontaneous haemorrhage will not occur, dental extractions may be performed as it is unlikely that they will be followed by excessive bleeding.

Table 5 Relation of factor deficiency and clinical disease

Factors	Other names	Deficiency disease
Factor I	Fibrinogen	Hypofibrinogenaemia
Factor II	Prothrombin	Hypoprothrombinaemia
Factor III	Thromboplastin	
Factor IV	Calcium ions	
Factor V	Proaccelerin	Factor V deficiency
Factor VI	Does not exist	
Factor VII	Proconvertin	Factor VII deficiency
Factor VIII	Antihaemophilic factor	Haemophilia A
Factor IX	{ Christmas factor Plasma thromboplastin component (PTC)	Haemophilia B Christmas disease
Factor X	Stuart factor	Stuart factor deficiency
Factor XI	Plasma thromboplastin antecedent (PTA)	PTA deficiency
Factor XII	Hageman factor	Hageman factor deficiency
Factor XIII	Fibrin stabilising factor (FSF)	FSF deficiency

Investigation of post-extraction haemorrhage

A history of excessive bleeding is most commonly due to local factors, but particular attention should be paid to those who on several occasions have undergone repeated attempts to arrest post-extraction or other haemorrhage. These need careful investigation to eliminate a possible systemic cause. Petechial haemorrhage (purpura) and bruising are typical of generalised vascular damage and platelet inadequacy, but not of clotting disorders. Recurrent haemarthrosis is suggestive of haemophilia A and B, but not of platelet or vascular disorders. The family history is important as many of the conditions are hereditary.

Wherever the surgeon's suspicions are aroused the patient must be referred to a haematologist for full investigation before operation, as only in the laboratory can the diagnosis be made.

Treatment

Patients with systemic haemorrhagic disease should be admitted to hospital for surgery and treated in conjunction with a haematologist.

In vascular disorders management depends on local measures and arranging for blood to be available for transfusion should *the loss* make this necessary.

In platelet disorders secondary to other diseases the cause must be dealt with first. Patients with idiopathic thrombocytopenia may be given steroid therapy to raise the platelet count or pre-operative platelet infusions.

In clotting disorders the essential treatment is to replace the missing factor. For haemophilia A and Von Willebrand's disease factor VIII is available and given by intravenous injection. For patients with mild disease D.D.A.V.P. (desmopressin) will raise the patient's endogenous factor VIII. Tranexamic acid is an antifibrinolytic agent used to prevent the destruction of clots and is given for ten days commencing one day pre-operatively.

Choice of anaesthetic. In vascular and platelet disorders either a general or local anaesthetic is satisfactory.

In clotting disorders caution should be used with regard to local anaesthesia, particularly inferior dental and posterior superior dental blocks, owing to the danger of producing a large haematoma which could endanger the airway. Injections down the periodontal membrane may provide adequate anaesthesia for extraction of teeth. General anaesthesia is sometimes indicated and should be administered by an experienced anaesthetist.

Local dental measures. These include oral prophylaxis, improving oral hygiene and *conservation procedures to reduce the number of extractions*. The operation is planned and executed to cause minimal trauma and it is wise to extract teeth from only one quadrant of the mouth at any time. In the local arrest of haemorrhage, sutures should not be used in patients with clotting defects as bleeding may continue into the tissue spaces particularly in the floor of the mouth.

Respiratory disorders

Bronchitis

This common condition is an acute or chronic inflammation of the mucosa lining the bronchi, which has seasonal exacerbations and is often associated with other conditions, particularly upper respiratory tract infections and bronchiectasis.

All patients suffering from bronchitis and bronchiectasis are best treated under local anaesthesia. Where a general anaesthetic is required they should be assessed by a specialist anaesthetist well beforehand, as many are improved by medical preparation including antibiotics, physiotherapy, and breathing exercises.

Asthma

In asthma there are intermittent attacks of bronchospasm complicated by the secretion of thick mucus and mucosal swelling. It is believed to be an allergic disease, and the use of allergenic substances (e.g. penicillin) is best avoided. Some patients are under treatment with bronchodilators in the form of an inhaler whilst others may use a corticosteroid aerosol inhaler. General anaesthesia, though not generally contraindicated, should be administered by a specialist anaesthetist.

In acute attacks the airway must be maintained, and in this respect asthmatic patients breathe more easily when upright. To relieve spasm inhalation of the bronchodilator should help, but if this fails, hydrocortisone should be administered intravenously.

Infectious diseases

The dental surgeon and staff are at risk from acquiring infections from patients. These include the common cold, xanthemata, tuberculosis, cytomegalovirus, herpes, hepatitis and human immune deficiency virus (H.I.V). Precautions must be taken to avoid infection of the surgical team as well as preventing cross-infection between patients.

Viral hepatitis

Several viruses cause hepatitis. Those of importance are virus A, B and C (non-A, non-B). Virus A is transmitted by faecal contamination of food and water and has an incubation period of thirty days. The B virus is transmitted by blood or serum, the incubation period being about one hundred days. The virus of hepatitis C has recently been identified and transmission is by blood and serum. Chronic carriers of the hepatitis B – e antigen must be regarded as highly infectious. A very careful operative technique and system for sterilisation of instruments is required to protect surgery staff and other patients. All staff should be advised to be immunised against the hepatitis B virus as unrecognised carriers of the antigen may present for treatment.

Human Immune Deficiency Virus (H.I.V)

The retrovirus H.I.V. was recognised in 1980 and is transmitted by blood and semen, although it has been isolated from other body fluids. A test for specific antibodies to H.I.V. is available and its presence indicates that the patient can transmit the disease. Whilst some individuals will be aware of their status others may be H.I.V.-positive unknowingly. Since the numbers of affected people is increasing it is wise for precautions to be taken during the treatment of *all* patients, so that there is no risk of infection to the surgical team or other patients. Fortunately the virus is easily inactivated by heat or by the use of hypochlorite.

Those who are H.I.V.-positive are at risk of developing acquired immune deficiency syndrome (AIDS), but the incubation period is unknown. These patients have a compromised cell-mediated immune response and develop opportunistic infections. In the oral cavity candidosis, hairy leukoplakia and Kaposi's sarcoma are manifestations of Acquired Immune Deficiency Syndrome. Patients who develop AIDS should be referred to hospital for treatment.

Epilepsy

Epilepsy is a disease of the central nervous system in which there is a paroxysmal electrochemical disturbance. This may result in fits of two types. 'Petit mal' is of a minor character in which, without warning, the patient loses consciousness for a few seconds, but seldom falls or has convulsions. 'Grand mal' is characterised by generalised convulsions and loss of consciousness, and is sometimes heralded by the so-called 'aura', or peculiar sensation, which warns the patient of an impending attack. During the fit the pulse and blood pressure remain normal but muscle contractions may affect respiration causing cyanosis and the tongue may be bitten if not protected.

Prevention is by avoiding excitement and ensuring that patients take their normal dose of anticonvulsant drugs. Where a fit occurs the airway is maintained and the patient turned onto his side and protected from injury. Wooden wedges are inserted between the teeth bilaterally to safeguard the tongue, dentures are removed and the mouth sucked out. Recovery occurs slowly without treatment if the patient is left quietly to regain consciousness. The exception is status epilepticus, where one fit follows another in rapid succession; this may be treated by a slow intravenous injection of diazepam.

Systemic diseases of bone

These conditions affect the dental surgeon in four ways. Difficulties in extraction of teeth may be encountered due to hypercementosis (osteitis deformans—'Paget's disease') or sclerosis of bone (osteopetrosis, acromegaly).

The bone may be fragile, leading to fracture even though minimal force is used during operations (osteogenesis imperfecta). The incidence of post-operative infection is increased (osteitis deformans) and there may be risk of causing an exacerbation of the disease (fibrous dysplasia) or a malignant change in the bone (osteitis deformans).

The successful treatment of these patients lies in a correct diagnosis of the condition followed by careful pre-operative preparation.

Depressive illness

Tricyclic antidepressant drugs which are used in treating depressive illness interact with adrenalin to cause hypertension. Patients on these drugs should not be given adrenalin, but felyipressin can safely be used as a vasoconstrictor. Monoamine oxidase inhibitors are sometimes given for depression. They potentiate the action of many drugs including barbiturates and adrenalin, the effect lasting for two weeks after stopping the drug.

Further reading

Rees, P. J. and Trounce, J. R. (1988), *A New Short Textbook of Medicine*. Edward Arnold, London.

Thomson, Jean (1985), *Blood Coagulation and Haemostasis: A Practical Guide*, 3rd edn. Churchill Livingstone, Edinburgh.

Walter, J. B. and Israel, M. S. (1987), *General Pathology*, 6th edn. Churchill Livingstone, Edinburgh.

Walton, John G., Thompson, J. W. and Seymour, R. A. (1989), *Textbook of Dental Pharmacology and Theurapeutics*. Oxford University Press, Oxford.

iv Emergencies in oral surgery

Any emergency can be terrifying if it occurs without warning and the dental surgeon is unprepared. The element of surprise can be reduced by completing careful histories and investigations to identify the poor-risk patients and enlisting the help of a physician to prepare them for operation. Only by study and experience will the dental surgeon acquire the ability to diagnose and treat quickly those emergencies that may arise. He may be gravely handicapped if the essential drugs and instruments are not readily to hand or if his assistants are untrained.

All essential items for resuscitation should be kept in a special container, the drugs clearly labelled with their name, strength of the solution or tablet, the dose, method of administration and expiry date. Instruments such as hypodermic syringes are stored, ready sterilised, in sealed containers. Oxygen and suction should always be available. Usually two assistants are required, one to help with the patient and one free to fetch and carry. The telephone numbers of the ambulance, fire service, local hospital and the nearest medical practitioners should be readily available.

All these preparations are useless if the team is not regularly rehearsed by mock emergency drills so that each unhesitatingly knows the part he has to play. Emergencies may arise as an acute phase of a known medical condition; this group has been discussed in Chapter III. Others occur as a result of surgical procedures (Chapter VII) or without previous history, and these are described here.

Fainting

This is the commonest emergency seen by the dentist as it is often precipitated by the emotional disturbances or pain associated with surgical procedures. In fainting a general peripheral vasodilatation, particularly in the muscles, cause cerebral ischaemia, with loss of consciousness.

Signs and symptoms. These are pallor, nausea, dizziness, and a cold sweat, which if ignored are followed by loss of consciousness. The blood pressure falls, the pulse rate remains normal but the volume is weak and thready. The pupils are dilated and rolled up.

Treatment. This consists in promply lying the patient down in the supine position with the head lower than the heart and the feet well up. The airway is checked, dentures are removed, the jaw is drawn forward and tight clothing is loosened. Verbal communication with the patient is important both as a measure of reassurance and to ascertain their level of consciousness. Starved patients, who are not diabetics, should be given a glucose drink. This treatment is usually successful but should the fall in blood pressure persist oxygen is given and a physician must be consulted.

Anaphylaxis

Anaphylaxis is an acute hypersensitivity reaction to substances to which the patient has been previously sensitised. These may be sera, local anaesthetic solutions, penicillin or other allergenic substances. Prevention is best effected by ensuring that all those with a history of allergy, asthma or hay fever do not receive drugs known to cause such reactions, particularly by injection.

Signs and symptoms. These usually begin within half an hour of introducing the foreign substance. The reaction is characterised by urticaria, particularly at the site of injection, by cyanosis, and dyspnoea due to bronchospasm and oedema, by sweating and a general feeling of faintness. These are accompanied by a raised pulse, a fall in blood pressure and the onset of circulatory collapse and death.

Treatment. This consists in laying the patient down with their feet well up, maintaining the airway and injecting *at once* 0.5 – 1 ml of adrenaline 1 : 1,000 solution by intramuscular injection. This should raise the blood pressure and dilate the bronchi. Where the hypotension persists, a further dose ten minutes later using a different limb is given. Antihistamine (chlorpheniramine) given by slow intravenous injection may be helpful. The blood pressure is checked repeatedly and if hypotension is persistent an intravenous saline drip may be required.

Hypoglycaemic shock. See page 21.

Acute adrenal insufficiency. See page 20.

Surgical shock

This rarely occurs following oral surgical procedures unless the operation is very prolonged or is accompanied by excessive blood loss. Following severe injury or long continued post-extraction haemorrhage patients may be seen in a state of shock and require urgent treatment. Surgical shock is a result of fluid loss (either serum from burns or blood from open or closed wounds). In closed wounds blood and plasma may bleed from the vessels into the tissue spaces, It is believed that if the initial loss is over one litre or one-quarter of the blood volume of six litres, this is more than can be compensated for by the general vasoconstriction. Where this is not replaced, then a vicious circle is set up in which the falling blood pressure and the general vasoconstriction cause oxygen lack in the tissues and an increased permeability of the capillaries with still further loss of fluid into the tissues.

Signs and symptoms. The patient is typically cold, sweating and pale or cyanosed. There is often gasping respiration or air hunger. In the limbs the degree of swelling in closed injuries gives some indication of the fluid loss into the tissues, but this is of little use in facial injuries. The pulse is rapid and the blood pressure low.

Treatment. Prompt and energetic measures in good time are necessary. First, arrest of haemorrhage must be undertaken to prevent further loss, whilst an assistant takes and charts pulse and blood pressure readings at short intervals (fifteen minutes). In the mildly shocked patient fluids, such as warm, sweet tea may be given by mouth if no operation is envisaged in the next six hours, and no abdominal injury is present. A rising pulse rate and a falling blood pressure is an ominous sign. A patient with a pulse rate persistently over 100, and systolic blood pressure of under 100 mm (13.3 KPa), almost certainly requires transfusion and blood should be taken for grouping and cross matching. This should be done early, and whenever there is doubt a slow saline or plasma substitute (e.g. dextran) drip started before the veins collapse.

A choice must be made whether to give saline or plasma to replace fluid, or whole blood which will raise the circulating haemoglobin as well. Unfortunately, haemoglobin estimations are of little use in the acute phase owing to the haemoconcentration which usually occurs. The decision is made from the history or observation of the actual blood loss from open or closed wounds but whichever is given the haemoglobin level must be checked to avoid haemoconcentration or haemodilution.

The circulation to the head is improved by raising the foot of the bed. In cyanosed patients oxygen may be administered. Warmth should be applied with blankets to keep the patient in an environmental temperature of 32°C. No other heating devices, which might cause furthr peripheral vasodilation, should be used.

Relief of pain may be achieved by temporarily splinting or supporting fractures, by dressing open wounds and by prescribing analgesics.

Acute respiratory obstruction and arrest

This may occur during dental operations under inhalation general anaesthetic due to the inhalation of vomit or a foreign body if the oropharynx is inadequately packed. A second cause is an acute inflammatory swelling of the neck.

Signs and symptoms. The patient stops breathing and though a few jerky respiratory movements are made he is unable to inflate his lungs. The face and neck rapidly become very congested and cyanosed.

Treatment. Immediately the patient becomes anoxic the surgeon should stop the operation, draw the tongue forward, and reduce any pressure from the pack or the chin which might occlude the airway, and suck out any debris in the mouth or oropharynx. Meanwhile the anaesthetist searches for any cause of anoxia such as failure of the oxygen supply, obstruction in the tubes of the anaesthetic apparatus, excessive formation of mucus in the respiratory tract, vomiting behind the pack, or swelling of the throat and neck. The dental surgeon should *silently* observe that each has been investigated, but if one is overlooked he should draw attention to it. He should call for the tracheostomy set and can usefully take the pulse in case cardiac arrest should supervene. The passing of an endotracheal tube will usually restore the airway; however intubation may not be possible, making it necessary to make an opening into the trachea below the obstruction. This may be achieved by cricothyroid puncture or by tracheostomy.

Cricothyroid puncture. A cricothyroid needle, specially designed for the purpose, can be used to pierce the skin and cricothyroid membrane and form a passage for air. However this, though relatively simple to do, can only be considered a temporary expedient.

Emergency tracheostomy. The landmarks for this operation are the cricoid cartilage and the midline of the neck, which may be difficult to identify owing to the gross congestion. The head is held firmly with the neck fully extended over a sandbag so as to bring the trachea as near the surface as possible. The thumb and middle fingers of the left hand palpate and identify the cricoid cartilage which they then grasp throughout the operation (Fig. 1).

The incision is made through all the superficial tissues from the thyroid notch to a point one centimetre above the sternal notch. There will be much bleeding due to congestion, but if the incision is in the midline, there is no danger. The index finger of the left hand is placed in the wound to identify and protect the cricoid cartilage. The incision is deepened on to the trachea,

Fig. 1 Incision for emergency tracheostomy. Note the position of the thumb, the second finger and major vessels. The first finger has been omitted but enters the wound and palpates the lower border of the cricoid. The inset shows a support under the shoulders to put the neck on full extension.

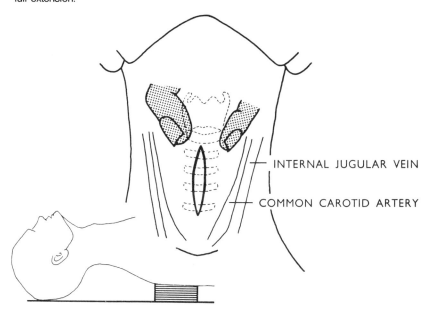

INTERNAL JUGULAR VEIN

COMMON CAROTID ARTERY

the thyroid isthmus is divided if necessary. The second and third tracheal rings are incised. To protect the posterior tracheal wall, all but the last centimetre of the scalpel blade is guarded by gauze or the fingers. The scalpel is withdrawn and the tracheal incision dilated with the handle. Where no introducer or tracheostomy tube is available any rubber tube of about half a centimetre diameter will serve to maintain the airway. Care must be taken that the tube is not accidentally put into the tissues at either side of the trachea. Once the tube is held firmly in place to prevent it displacing into the trachea the emergency is over and respirations should restart and bleeding may be controlled. As soon as possible the patient is put under the care of an otorhinolaryngologist.

Coronary heart disease. See page 23.

Cardiac arrest

Cardiac arrest is of two kinds, cardiac asystole in which the heart is motionless, and ventricular fibrillation in which the action of the heart though present is uncoordinated and ineffective so that circulation is not maintained. The chief predisposing cause is cardiovascular disease and the immediate exciting factors are anoxia, or an overdose of drugs particularly the anaesthetic agent, and vagal stimulation.

Signs and symptoms. The pulse is absent in the carotid and other major arteries, the blood pressure cannot be recorded and bleeding stops from the operation wound. The respirations cease and the pupils are widely dilated and fixed.

Treatment. Cardiac massage is the only accepted remedy and every dental surgeon must be prepared to attempt it *without delay*; three minutes is the limit of anoxia that the brain will tolerate before irreversible changes take place. The anaesthetist (or the surgeon's assistant if the arrest occurs under local anaesthetic) lays the patient flat and maintains a clear airway by removing all obstructions, drawing the tongue forward and pushing the jaw forward by pressing at the angles. He insufflates the lungs, preferably using oxygen through an endotracheal tube. Where these are not available mouth-to-mouth breathing may be used.

Mouth to mouth respiration. After clearing the mouth and pharynx of debris and fluids, the neck is extended by flexing the head dorsally. The chin is drawn forward by grasping the lower jaw with one hand, whilst the other pinches the nostrils to seal them. The operator's wide open mouth is applied to the patient's (or an airway) to form an airtight seal. Air is then exhaled into the patient's mouth with sufficient force and volume to expand his lungs. The chest should be seen to rise and fall between each breath. This is repeated twelve to eighteen times a minute. Where available a Brook airway or Laerdal pocket mask will facilitate artificial respiration.

Cardiac massage. The surgeon strips the patient's chest of all clothing preparatory to giving cardiac massage. External cardiac massage is given by lying the patient flat on a firm surface. The operator kneels beside him and places the palm of one hand on the sternum just above the xiphisternum. The other hand is laid over the first. The arms are kept straight and with the whole weight of the body the sternum is depressed about 5 cm downwards (Fig. 2). In this way the heart is compressed between the sternum and the vertebral column and the ventricles empty (Fig. 3). Pressure is reapplied in this way sixty to eighty times a minute and if done satisfactorily a circulation can be maintained with a recordable blood pressure. In children the pressure should be less and applied to the middle of the sternum at a rate of one hundred times a minute.

To allow effective ventilation, insufflation is performed at every fifth *upstroke* of cardiac massage. Where one individual is faced with both tasks he will similarly insufflate the lungs between each fifteen strokes of cardiac massage.

Fig. 2 External cardiac massage. Note how 'heels' of the hands are used to press on the sternum whilst the assistant supports the mandible and gives artificial respiration through the Brook airway.

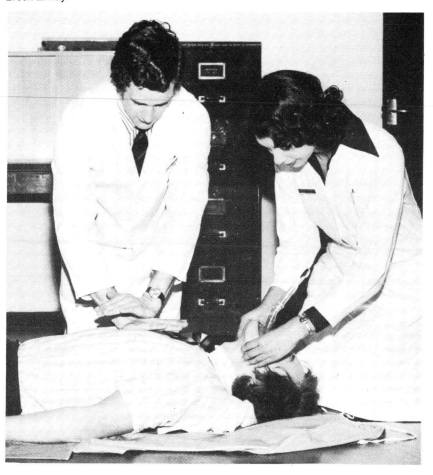

Fig. 3 (a) Shows the relationship of the heart to the sternum and ribs. (b) Shows how pressure on the xiphisternum compresses the heart between the sternum and the vertebral column.

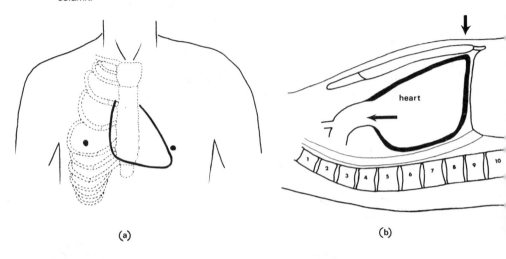

(a) (b)

About ten minutes of this exercise is as much as one person can manage but massage should normally be continued till the heart starts beating normally or expert help, with a defibrillator, is available.

Cerebral vascular accidents

An acute cerebral vascular accident may occur as a result of rupture, thrombosis or embolism in a cerebral vessel.

Signs and symptoms. These will obviously vary widely according to the size and the site of the vessels involved. The following are typical of most such catastrophies. The onset is sudden but not all patients go into coma. The face is flushed or cyanosed, breathing slow and stertorous and the pulse is slow and bounding. Hemiplegia and changes in reactions of the pupils are frequently present. In conscious patients the speech is often affected.

Treatment. This consists of maintaining the airway and giving oxygen. The patient should be kept quiet and not moved till seen by a physician.

Death in the surgery or operating theatre

When death occurs the dental surgeon should tell the patient's relatives and general medical practitioner, speaking to the relatives personally. The coroner must be notified as soon as possible of the name and address of the deceased and the time and circumstances of the death. A written report must be submitted to the coroner's clerk within twenty-four hours. The dental surgeon may attend the post-mortem if it is ordered and it is advisable to do so. He may be directed, by the coroner, to attend the inquest and give evidence. It is wise in the case of such a calamity to seek the advice of a medical protection society before writing the report or attending the post-mortem or inquest.

Further reading

Frame, J. H. (1972), 'An emergency drug cabinet for use in general dental practice', *Brit. Dent. J.*, **132**, 363.
Marsden, A. K. (1989), 'Basic life support', *Brit. Med. J.*, **299**, 442.
Norris, W. and Campbell, D. (1985), *Anaesthetics, Resuscitation and Intensive care*, 6th edn. Churchill Livingstone, Edinburgh.

v Prescribing for certain common conditions or needs in oral surgery

Prescribing

The prescription must contain instructions to the pharmacist for preparing the medicine and to the patient for taking it. They are written in ink according to an accepted form. Today it is generally agreed that plain English is far preferable to a bastardised attempt at the classics and further that all figures should be clearly expressed in arabic numerals and the quantities in grammes.

Before writing a prescription it is important always to consider the following points.

The pharmacological action of the drug

At no time should any drug be prescribed if its action is not clearly understood. In this respect side-effects should be carefully considered. The British National Formulary published twice-yearly gives a good outline of actions and side effects and should be consulted if there is any doubt about the suitability of a particular drug. It is a good principle to have a repertoire of a few well-tried drugs which meet the needs of day-to-day practice, and to understand them well, rather than to experiment with a wide range.

Contraindications and incompatibility of drugs

In certain medical conditions some drugs are contraindicated, for example sulphonamides in chronic renal disease. Incompatibility of drugs occasionally arises, though it should be borne in mind, but a more common and dangerous complication is an anaphylactic reaction in those patients sensitive to a drug (e.g. penicillin). It is therefore important to question the patient carefully about previous treatment and reaction and any history of urticaria or asthma, as sufferers from these conditions seem more likely to be sensitive. Wherever there is doubt about the proposed drug an alternative should be used.

Dosage

Today the formularies make it unnecessary to give details of the constituent parts of medicines, but the correct title and strength of the drug, together with the four 'Hows', must be clearly stated:

How much of the drug is to be taken in each individual dose.

How often it is to be taken, expressed as the number of doses in each twenty-four hours and the interval between each.

How long the course is to run, expressed in days, so that it is not continued overlong or stopped before the clinician thinks fit.

How it is to be administered, by mouth, intramuscularly, etc.

The British National Formularies give suggested doses of accepted remedies for adults and children, to which reference must be made before prescribing. Excretion of drugs in the elderly may be slow and particular care is needed when prescribing drugs for them.

The importance of giving adequate doses for a specific purpose cannot be overstressed. Low doses must be avoided if drug therapy is to be effective.

An example of a prescription is shown below

Date

    R$_x$ 250 mg phenoxymethyl penicillin tablets
              Send 20 (twenty)
              Label 1 tablet orally for 5 days.

                              Signature

Method of administration

By mouth. This route is the most popular and the least upsetting to the patient. Its chief disadvantage is that the rate of absorption from the gut cannot be forecast for any individual. It may be rapid, delayed, or not occur at all. The substance may be destroyed or altered by the digestive juices. Other complications may be caused by side effects on the alimentary tract and its bacterial flora.

By injection. Drugs can be injected subcutaneously, intramuscularly or intravenously.

For the first two a hypodermic needle 21 G on an aspirating syringe is used to draw up the drug and to give the injection. The skin is cleansed with spirit. Before the drug is injected aspiration is performed to ensure the needle is not in a blood vessel.

Subcutaneous injection. The needle is passed into the subcutaneous tissues through a fold of loose skin which has been pinched up between finger and thumb to separate it from the underlying tissues.

Intramuscular injection. The safest site is into the vastus lateralis muscle, that is into the lateral aspect of the middle third of the thigh. The skin is tensed with the left hand and the needle inserted at an angle of 90° through the skin into the muscle. The buttock should not be used lest the sciatic nerve be damaged.

Intravenous injection. An aspirating syringe with a 23 G bore needle is used. An appropriate vein is chosen preferably on the hand or forearm which should be visible and reasonably straight. It is artificially distended by manual compression or tourniquet above the site, which is then cleaned with spirit. The vein is held in place by slight traction distal to the vessel. The needle is introduced through the skin and into the vein at an angle under 45°. Successful entry is confirmed by a back flow of blood into the syringe. The tourniquet is released and the injection may be given.

Pre-operative medication

In premedication for operation there are two chief considerations, firstly the sedation of the patient to allay apprehension, and secondly the inhibition of the oral and respiratory tract secretions before general anaesthesia. There is an unfortunate tendency to reserve premedication for those patients treated in hospital and particularly those receiving a general anaesthetic. It is equally important to alleviate apprehension in the out-patient, whatever the anaesthetic proposed. Those drugs which depress the vital centres must not be given unless adequate post-operative facilities are available, the patient is accompanied, and has no car to drive home. Premedication should start the night before operation to ensure a good night's sleep. Where the patient is to have a general anaesthetic the anaesthetist should be consulted as to which drugs and dosages he prefers. Suggested drugs and doses are shown below.

Night before operation　for both in- and out-patients

For sedation

Hypnotics
P.o.M. Nitrazepam tablets B.N.F.
　Adults 5 mg
　30 mins before retiring
　　　or
P.o.M. Temazepam tablets B.N.F.
　Adults 10 mg
　　immediately before retiring
　　　or
P.o.M. Chloral Mixture B.N.F.
　Adults 5–20 mL
　Children 1–5 years 2.5–5 mL
　　　6–12 years 5–10 mL

Anxiolytics
P.o.M. Diazepam B.N.F.
　Adults 5 mg

P.o.M. Diazepam elixir
　2 mg in 5 mL of elixir
　Children 1–5 year, 1.25 mL
　　　6–12 years, 2.5 mL

Preoperatively

Outpatient

For sedation
P.o.M. Diazepam tablets B.N.F.
　5 mg 1 hour pre-operatively

Inpatient

For sedation
P.o.M. Papaveretum inj. B.N.F.
　0.5–1 mL subcutaneously 1 hour
　　pre-operatively
　　　or
P.o.M. Lorazepam – 2–4 mg orally 2 hours
　　pre-operatively
　　　or
For children over 2 years
P.o.M. Trimeprazine Tartrate
　2 mg per kg body weight 2 hours
　　pre-operatively

To inhibit secretions

P.o.M. Atropine sulphate B.N.F.
　Adults 300–600 mg
　　intramuscular injection
　　1 hour pre-operatively

P.o.M.: Prescription-only medicine
B.N.F.: British National Formulary

A warning must be issued about over-sedation of patients admitted for oral surgery. Following general anaesthesia the patient should regain consciousness as soon as possible and this is especially desirable where there is trismus or where intermaxillary fixation is in place. Over-sedation in conjunction with a short anaesthetic may mean that the premedicant drug is still acting during the recovery period. This can delay the patient's return to full consciousness and the control of his airway. Where this could be serious premedication with only atropine sulphate (1 mg) has much to commend it.

Sedation and local anaesthesia

Intravenous sedation

Sedative drugs, particularly the benzodiazepines, have been used on nervous out-patients to assist their management under local anaesthesia. The dosage is such to produce light sedation with retention of pharyngeal reflexes. An emulsion preparation of Diazepam is currently popular as the complication of venous thrombosis post-operatively is low. Midazolam, a water-soluble Benzodiazepine, is also used but must be given in very low dosage to avoid respiratory depression (see B.N.F.). The usual technique is to bring the patient to the surgery prepared as for a general anaesthetic (Chapter II). With the patient lying supine a slow intravenous injection of Diazepam emulsion (5 mg in 1 mL) is given: 10–20 mg given over 2–4 minutes. The correct dosage has been given when drooping of the upper lid (ptosis) occurs and this half covers the pupils. This is known as Verrill's sign.

The local anaesthetic may then be injected and the operation commenced. It is important to realise that if the dose of diazepam is not carefully controlled the patient may lose consciousness and therefore continuous monitoring of the patient must be undertaken. Facilities for intubation and giving oxygen must be available.

After using this technique the patient cannot be considered fit to drive or handle machinery and requires to be accompanied home after a prolonged recovery period for all of which the dental surgeon must make provision.

Relative analgesia (inhalation sedation)

In this sedation technique nitrous oxide and oxygen are administered to the patient through a nose piece in a varying proportion which may range from 30–80% oxygen and 70–20% nitrous oxide. After inhalation of the mixture the patient should be relaxed and co-operative and where necessary can be given a local anaesthetic for the operative procedure. The patient should be prepared as for a general anaesthetic and similar arrangements made for his recovery.

Post-operative medication

Sedation

Hypnotics should be withheld after a general anaesthetic lest the unconscious state be prolonged and blood or mucus inhaled. Sedation for inability to sleep may be considered when the patient is fully 'round' and it is certain that post-operative bleeding has quite ceased, when Nitrazepam may be prescribed.

Analgesia

Patients sometimes complain of pain after oral surgery and should they do so, every effort must be made to find and treat the cause if the amount of pain seems inappropriate to the operative procedure. For mild pain one or two 300 mg tablets of dispersible aspirin are an effective analgesic but should not be given to children, patients with gastrointestinal problems, those on anticoagulant therapy or who have a bleeding diathesis. Paracetamol may be used as an alternative. For in-patients stronger analgesics may be given after consultation with the anaesthetist.

Sore lips

These are caused by the cheek retractors but their severity can be reduced by rubbing lanolin ointment into the lips before and after operation.

Sore throat

This may follow endotracheal intubation and packing of the throat with a dry pack. Where swallowing is difficult benzocaine compound lozenges may help before meals. Tracheitis and congestion of the nose can be helped by inhalations such as menthol and eucalyptus or benzoin.

Post-operative vomiting

This may be due to ingested blood and will cease once this has been ejected. Where vomiting or nausea persists it can frequently be stopped by giving the patient milk or alkaline drinks with glucose sipped very slowly. Where this fails an injection of Prochlorperazine 12.5 mg intramuscularly may be given.

Traumatic injuries

Analgesics and hypnotics

In traumatic injuries these may be prescribed as necessary provided the patient's reflexes are not so depressed that the airway may obstruct from bleeding or other causes. Similarly in a suspected head injury opiate analgesics or sedative drugs which could mask the signs of progressive intracranial pressure are to be avoided. All drugs given to patients must be carefully recorded and if they are transferred elsewhere the record sent with them.

Anti-infectives

Antibacterial substances are used prophylactically for a few days where there is a large haematoma which may become infected, and for a longer period where the deeper tissues, and particularly bone, have been contaminated.

In maxillary fractures which involve the cranial fossae with loss of cerebrospinal fluid through the nose, ears or pharynx, it is important to prevent intracranial infection by the use of an antibacterial which will cross the thecal barrier. This is satisfactorily achieved by giving sulphadimidine injection or tablets, initial dose 2 g, and thereafter 1 g six-hourly.

In all penetrating wounds contaminated with road dirt or soil the need for tetanus prophylaxis must be considered. In patients who have not been immunised or where five years have elapsed since the last reinforcing dose, 0.5 mL of absorbed tetanus vaccine should be given by intramuscular injection.

Infections

Today antibacterial drugs play an important part in the treatment of acute infections but they should not be considered a substitute for necessary surgery, though they are useful as a preparation or adjunct to such treatment. The object is to select for use the agent which gives the best therapeutic result with the minimal side effects. To do this the condition must be diagnosed, the causal organism isolated and its susceptibility to antibacterials tested *in vitro*. A course is then planned of sufficient concentration and duration that the formation of resistant strains is prevented. A satisfactory concentration in the blood is obtained by administering the drug parenterally wherever possible, and a high initial 'loading' dose is to be recommended. The drug should be changed if there is no response after forty-eight hours. As a guide, the dosage both in quantity and frequency is shown in Table 6. Generally the agents of choice are penicillin, amoxycillin, flucloxacillin and metronidazole. Where necessary, erythromycin, sulphonamides and clindamycin are used. Combinations of antibacterial drugs must be used with caution. Some combinations are effective, for example penicillin and metronidazole or penicillin and sulponamides. A warning is necessary that all these substances have side-reactions of importance which are mentioned in Table 6. Where the course is continued for a long time this risk is increased and careful supervision is important.

On many occasions, where it is not possible to ascertain the sensitivity of the organism, it may be essential to prescribe blind, but it should never be regarded as the method of choice. An antibiotic known to be effective in the type of infection under consideration should be used. In oral surgery

Table 6 Antibacterial agents. IM – Intramuscular injection.
All these drugs should be used for a minimum of three days to minimise the formation of resistant strains.

Antibacterial agent and administration	Action and organism affected	Maintenance			Side-effects	Prevention and treatment of side-effects
		Initial dose	Dose	Frequency in hours		
Penicillin Benzyl penicillin (IM)	*Bactericidal* Gram positive cocci Gram negative cocci	600 mg	300 mg	6		Careful history. If any doubt do *not* use again. Treatment see Chapter IV.
Procaine penicillin (IM)	Gram positive bacilli	600 mg	600 mg	12	Anaphylaxis Skin rashes	
Phenoxymethyl penicillin (orally)	Spirochaetes	500 mg	250 mg	6		
Amoxycillin (orally)	Gram positive orgs. Gram negative orgs.	500 mg	250 mg	8		
Flucloxacillin (orally)	Pencillinase- producing Staphylococci	500 mg	250 mg	6		
Cephalosporins (orally)	*Bactericidal* Staphylococci Streptococci Some anaerobic bacteria	500 mg	250 mg	6	Hypersensitivity	Careful history. Do not use in those allergic to penicillin

Drug (route)	Spectrum	Dose	Dose		Side effects	Notes
Metronidazole (orally)	Anaerobic bacteria	400 mg	400 mg	8	Nausea and headaches with alcohol. Potentiates some antigoagulants	Avoid alcohol. Do not use in pregnancy.
Erythromycin (orally)	Gram positive cocci Gram positive bacilli	500 mg	250 mg	6	Diarrhoea	If diarrhoea occurs stop drug.
Sulphadimidine (orally or IM)	*Bacteriostatic* Gram positive cocci Gram negative cocci Gram negative bacilli	1–2 g (oral) 1–2 g (IM)	1 g (oral) 1 g (IM)	4 4	Crystalluria, renal pain, haematuria and oliguria Hypersensitivity reactions vary from a rash to aplastic anaemia	Use for less than eight days. Plenty of fluids by mouth. Keep urine alkaline. Stop drug if symptoms occur, never use the drug again.

this is commonly penicillin, but if there is no response after forty-eight hours another antibacterial should be selected.

Medication of packs for sockets

It is often necessary to dress bone cavities after oral surgery. Many admirable bland substances spread on gauze such as acriflavine emulsion, vaseline, or liquid paraffin unfortunately rapidly grow foul in the mouth and require changing frequently.

The two medicaments most frequently used on ribbon gauze are bismuth, iodoform and paraffin paste (B.I.P.P.) or Whitehead's varnish (iodoform 200 g, benzoin 200 g, storax 150 g, balsam of tolu 100 g in ether to 2 l). B.I.P.P. may give rise to toxic symptoms from absorption of the bismuth but this is most unusual on small packs in sockets though it may occur if used on large packs in big cavities. Whitehead's varnish contains iodoform and patients may be sensitive to this, but it is otherwise safe and widely used.

Adverse drug reactions

Occasionally a patient will report an unexpected adverse reaction to a drug or medicament. In an attempt to identify such problems at an early stage, a system of individual reporting of occurrences has been developed. The Committee on Safety of Medicines (C.S.M.) collates the information and suitable forms for reporting will be found in the British National Formulary.

Further reading

British National Formulary, current edition (produced biannually), Pharmaceutical Press, London.

Data Sheet Compendium, current edition (produced annually). Datapharm, London.

Laurence, D. R., ed. P. N. Bennett (1987), *Clinical Pharmacology*, 6th edn. Churchill Livingstone, Edinburgh.

VI The operating room, instruments and the surgical team

This chapter discusses the dental surgery or theatre, the instruments for oral surgical operations and the preparation of the surgical team.

The operating room

The operating room both in hospital and general dental practice should be of simple design, the walls and furniture of materials easy to clean and the equipment normally required accommodated without overcrowding.

It should be well ventilated and kept at an even temperature of 18–21 °C, without undue humidity. In hospital theatres this is best done by positive pressure air-conditioning which also prevents contamination from the outside atmosphere. Next door to the operating room there should be a central recovery room with experienced nursing staff where the patient may recover on a couch or trolley within easy reach of surgeon and anaesthetist until both are satisfied that he is fit to return to the ward or to go home.

Equipment

Light. The light source should provide adequate illumination without production of heat, and be easily adjusted to shine into the mouth. A headlamp or fibre light attached to a handpiece are recommended for operations involving the palate or deep cavities such as cysts or the antrum.

Suction apparatus. No procedure however minor, particularly under general anaesthesia, should be attempted without suction apparatus. This must be tested before the operation starts and whenever possible as alternative form of suction should be available in case of breakdown. Electrical apparatus is very powerful but does occasionally fail. Suction from the water supply is very effective, simple, trouble-free and economical, and is ideally suited to the dental surgery. Compressed air can also provide powerful suction in a similar way. Whichever method is used a catchment bottle must be included in the circuit so that if roots are lost the bottle may be searched.

Radiographic viewing box. This should be so placed that the dental surgeon can see it without moving from the dental chair or operating table. It should incorporate a spotlight.

The dental engine. Though the conventional dental handpiece can be sterilised, its attachment to the dental electric engine or air motor presents a problem. The surgeon may be contaminated from the cable drive unless these are covered with a sterile sleeve. Alternatively, sterilisable surgical motors and handpieces are available, but due to their high cost these are usually only found in hospital practice. For the clean and rapid cutting of the bone without overheating it is necessary that the bur be washed by a continuous stream of sterile water. Handpieces with an integral irrigation system are available and provide automatic irrigation of the bur. The air-rota may be used for oral surgery if it can be sterilised satisfactorily and there is no danger of blowing air or oil into the wound. The chief disadvantage is a lack of 'feel' owing to the ease with which it cuts both tooth and bone so that special care is needed to avoid over-cutting.

The dental chair. This should be of a design in which the patient can lie flat and the operator may work seated as this is the position of choice. The light, dental engine and suction should be sufficiently adjustable that they can be used with a supine patient from either right or left side.

Electrical equipment. Where this is to be used in the presence of anaesthetic vapours which may form explosive mixtures of gases, the equipment, particularly the dental engine, must be adequately sealed and earthed by a competent electrician to prevent sparking or a build-up of static electricity which might cause an explosion.

Instruments

The selection of hand instruments depends on the surgeon's preference. In the succeeding chapters instruments suitable for the various procedures are suggested. It is the surgeon's responsibility to check that all those he needs are readily available. They should be laid up on sterile towels on a trolley.

Care and maintenance of surgical instruments

The principles of care and maintenance are four: to clean the instruments thoroughly, to examine them for defects, to repair or discard those that are defective, and to sharpen all cutting edges.

Mechanical cleaning. Mucus and clotted blood may harbour and protect bacteria and make it impossible for steam to reach them. The first step in the process of sterilization is to scrub all instruments until clean with a brush under a running cold water tap. A bath agitated by ultrasonic vibrations produces a very high standard of cleanliness especially for hinged instruments and for suction tubes and heads. The latter should have cold water sucked through them immediately the operation is finished.

Cleaning also includes stripping down, cleaning and oiling all working machinery such as handpieces.

Examination for defects. Broken or bent instruments are put aside for repair or discarded. Hinges are tightened if necessary. Disposable items, burs, injection needles and scalpel blades are thrown away.

Fig. 4 Sharpening of instruments: (a) sandpaper disc for sharpening *outside* of forceps blade; (b) chisel held at the correct angle on the stone by a hone guide.

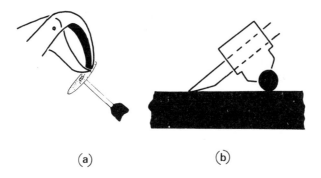

(a)   (b)

Sharpening. Stainless steel forceps and elevators are sharpened with a sandpaper disc in the dental handpiece (Fig. 4). It is only used on the outside of the blades, care being taken to maintain the angle of manufacture. There is a limit to how often these instruments can be sharpened before the working ends become too short.

Chisels have two bevels, one for grinding and one for sharpening. The angle for grinding is 20–25 degrees and for sharpening 35 degrees. Grinding is best left to an instrument technician and is done infrequently. Sharpening must be done each time the chisel is used. A hone guide will hold the bevelled side at the correct angle to the oil-stone when rubbing it up. Finally the flat side of the chisel is laid on the stone and rubbed two or three times to smooth the edge.

Sterilisation

Physical and chemical methods are both in use today. Physical methods include wet and dry heat, and gamma radiation (used commercially for sterilising packed instruments such as scalpel blades). Boiling water is no longer regarded as a safe method of sterilisation due to inherent problems with the length and control of the cycle.

Autoclaves use steam under pressure Some are high vacuum but all depend on downward displacement of air by steam. Steam at 2 kg cm^2 pressure gives a temperature of 134 °C which in three minutes will destroy all organisms and spores. It is the method of choice for dressing and towels, but they must be packed loosely to allow the steam to circulate. Blunting of instruments is due to oxidation which should not occur in a properly functioning autoclave, so that it can be safely used for sharp instruments. Vapour Phase Inhibitor (V.P.I.) paper can be used to wrap instruments such as burs which tend to rust if autoclaved. Handpieces must be cleaned and oiled before being placed in the autoclave. The oil must not become oxidised or lose its oily properties at high temperatures.

Dry heat is effective in ovens which have fans to ensure even heat distribution and a door-lock which prevents opening during the sterilising period. The cycle is much slower as it takes half an hour at $160\,^{\circ}$C to destroy organisms and spores. It may be used for sharp instruments and handpieces. Both autoclaves and hot-air sterilisers are made with controlled cycles which cannot be interrupted once started so that sterility of the instruments is ensured. The efficiency of the cycle must be checked periodically by the use of Brownes' tubes.

Chemical sterilising is not regarded favourably by bacteriologists as most of the solutions available are not considered reliable. Glutaraldehyde is effective against vegetative organisms and spores if the instruments are immersed in it for ten hours after which it must be washed off with sterile water, as it is irritant to tissues. Because of the length of the sterilising time and the irritant properties the use of glutaraldehyde is confined to those instruments which cannot be heat sterilised. Glutaraldehyde or hypochlorite solutions may be used to disinfect instruments potentially heavily contaminated with viruses (such as hepatitis) before these are cleaned and sterilised.

To sterilise with certainty autoclaving is the method of choice. Dry heat sterilising is the next best and only where both of these are impossible should chemical sterilising be considered.

Instruments packs

In hospital practice instruments are sterilised wrapped in paper containers. These are permeable to the steam in the autoclave and, providing the latter is of an evacuating type, are dry at the end of the cycle. Packs may be made up of one instrument or a complete layout for an operation including towels. They can be stored for up to six months ready for immediate use. The packs are duplicated according to the frequency with which they are used and may be prepared for local anaesthetic injections, flap preparation, suturing and so forth. This system is seldom available in general dental practice, making it necessary to sterilise and lay up instruments for each operation separately, though the hot air oven does make it possible to put groups of instruments in metal boxes which can then be stored sterile.

The surgical team

The surgeon

He is responsible for checking the identity if the patient and the nature of the operation to be performed, for the operation and for the surgical safety of the patient. His whole attention and effort must be devoted to this task and every assistance given him, that it may be completed safely and well. He is answerable for any procedure, planned or accidental, inflicted on the patient including those carried out by his assistants. He must be satisfied that all instruments swabs and packs are accounted for at the end of the operation.

All experienced staff realise the responsibility that rests on the surgeon and will overlook minor breaches of self-control that may occur. However, in an emergency, where speed and efficiency are wanted, an equable temperament and a firm determined manner will be more effective than any amount of histrionics.

The anaesthetist

The anaesthetist assesses the patient's fitness for general anaesthesia, chooses the anaesthetic agent, prescribes suitable premedication and administers the general anaesthetic. He will supervise the moving of the patient to and from the ward, and on and off the operating table, as well as his recovery from the anaesthetic and such post-anaesthetic complications as may arise.

During the operation he is responsible for the patient's airway, which should include packing of the throat and the removal of the pack after operation. He should continually assess the patient's general condition and report any deterioration to the surgeon, so that a mutual assessment of the situation can be made. As oral surgery procedures are seldom of a life-saving nature, the anaesthetist's opinion about the safety of the patient is accepted and surgical procedures planned or modified accordingly.

The surgeon's assistant

The dental surgeon's assistant in the hospital theatre is either a qualified colleague (house-surgeon or registrar) or a member of the nursing staff. In the dental surgery it will usually be a dental surgery assistant who, when trained by the dental surgeon, can be most efficient. The assistant will produce the patient's notes and radiographs and mount the latter correctly on the viewing box. She will then help with the preparation of the patient, by cleaning and towelling up the operation area and assembling the suction and other dental apparatus.

She will retract the tissues to give the surgeon the best possible access, clear fluid from the field of the operation with suction or swabs and remove solid debris with forceps. She assists with haemostasis by applying pressure or artery forceps, and with suturing by cutting the ends of the sutures.

The longer two people work together the greater will be the degree of team-work possible, with mutual benefit to all concerned. The surgeon will ask for further help in various special ways and, from qualified staff, advice based on previous experience, thereby extending their field of interest and responsibility.

The nursing staff

Before the operation begins the nursing staff will select and lay up those instruments, drugs and dressings they know to be necessary. They check the working of the dental engine, suction apparatus, and of all electrical appliances.

They follow the progress of the operation closely in order to anticipate the surgeon's needs and inspect and clean instruments, drawing attention to any that become broken or damaged. At the beginning and at the end of the operation they count all swabs, packs, dressings, instruments and needles, and tell the surgeon if any are missing before the patient leaves the theatre or the out-patient surgery.

Preparation of the surgical team

Those taking part in a surgical operation must be free from infection especially of the respiratory tract or skin which could be transmitted to the wound. All are responsible for their own safety and must develop a sensible routine which avoids skin or conjunctiva from being contaminated by blood or saliva from patients.

Dress.   All those entering a hospital operating theatre must change from their normal clothes into freshly laundered drill trousers and shirt, or dresses. This not only reduces the risk of contamination but is cooler and more comfortable, The hair is covered with a paper cap and a mask is worn over the mouth and nose. Safety glasses should be worn to avoid splashing of blood or irrigation fluid into the eyes. Shoes are changed for antistatic pumps, rubber boots or clogs used only in the theatre.

In the dental surgery a freshly laundered gown worn over everyday clothes is put on for each patient. A mask and protective glasses should be worn. The use of a cap is optional.

Scrubbing up.   Those who have to handle sterile instruments or dressings must undertake the ritual of 'scrubbing up'. The arms are bared to the elbow and all rings and watches removed. The hands and forearms are washed under a running tap, using an antiseptic detergent solution. They are well soaped and washed from the tips of the fingers up towards the elbow. The fingernails must be kept trimmed short for satisfactory cleansing which is done with a sterile scrubbing brush or nail scraper. At intervals, but not too frequently, the suds are rinsed away under the tap, being made to flow off at the elbow, not at the hands. This is continued for four minutes by the clock. The hands are then dried on a sterile towel by wiping from the hands up to the elbows. For minor procedures carried out in the dental surgery sterile gloves are put on and the operation commenced. For more extensive operations or where there is a risk of infection of staff and in theatre to conform with normal practice, a sterile gown and gloves are worn.

Gowning up.   The sterile gown is lifted from its container folded in such a way that if held correctly with both hands at its neck, it will unroll and fall with the sleeves hanging away from the operator. The arms are then placed in the sleeves and a second person standing behind draws the gown over the shoulders and fastens the tapes and belt at the back. The belt avoids billowing and rubbing of the gown and is an antistatic precaution.

The hands are now lightly dusted with powdered starch before drawing on the rubber gloves. These are taken from their envelope by the cuffs, which are folded down over the palms. The cuff of the right glove is held in the left hand and the right hand thrust in. The right hand then lifts the left glove by placing the fingers *under* the rolled cuff and the left hand is thrust in. The cuffs are turned back over the wrist to cover the sleeve (Fig. 5). In this way at no time will the hands have been in contact with outside of either gown or gloves. From this moment if any unsterilised object is touched the operator must gown up again.

Fig. 5 Gloving up. *Above left:* Holding right glove by cuff. *Above right:* Drawing on the right glove. *Below left:* Drawing on the left glove which is held under the turned-back cuff. *Below right:* Drawing the cuff over the sleeve.

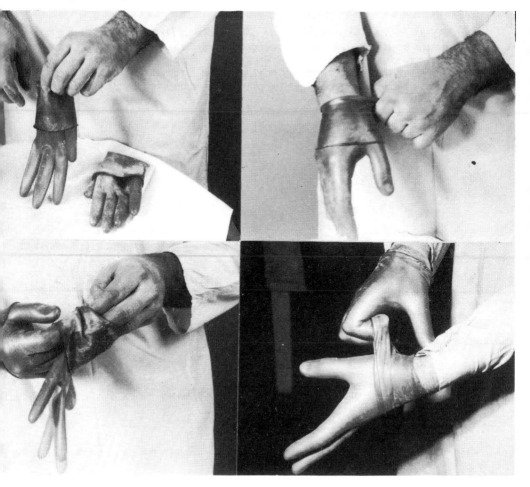

An alternative method has been introduced to reduce the risk of contamination of the outside of the gown or gloves. After gowning both hands remain covered by the sleeves. The left glove, with its fingers directed towards the elbow, is placed with the palm surface against the left sleeve. The cuff of the glove is grasped through the material by the thumb and fingers of the left hand. The right hand (through the gown material) grasps the outer part of the glove cuff and turns it over the sleeve of the gown. The glove is drawn onto the left hand by pulling glove and sleeve up the forearm (Fig. 6).

Preparation of the patient

In hospitals a label carrying the patient's name, address and hosptial number is attached to the wrist. The details should be checked against the patient's notes. A valid consent form must be available before the general anaesthetic is started. When local anaesthetic is being used mistaken idenity may be avoided by direct questioning of the patient.

Fig. 6 An alternative method of gloving up. *Above left:* Holding cuff of the left glove through the sleeve of the gown. *Above right:* Through the gown the right hand grasps the upper cuff of the left glove. *Lower left:* The left glove cuff being drawn over the gown by the right hand. The fingers on the right hand are shown for clarity but should be completely covered by the gown. *Lower right:* The gloved left hand drawing the right glove and gown upwards on the hand.

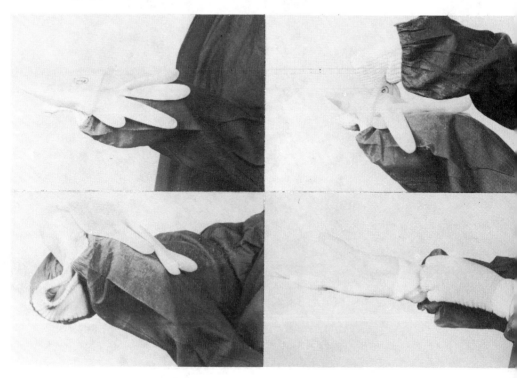

Fig. 7 Towelling up. *Left:* Cleaning the face. Note the sterile swab used for holding the face and protecting the eyes. *Right:* Two towels are placed beneath the head. The upper towel is used to cover the upper part of the face and the anaesthetic tube.

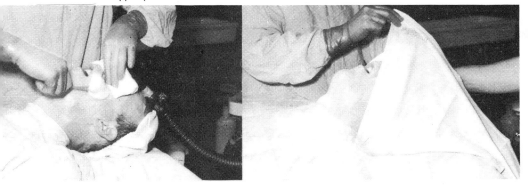

In theatre with the patient lying on the operating table, intubated and with the throat packed off, the surgeon checks his position on the table and has it adjusted if unsatisfactory. The operator then cleanses the site of operation, usually the mouth and surrounding skin, with a swab held in forceps and dipped in a clear detergent (chlorhexidine), care being taken to protect the eyes (Fig.7). The patient's body and head are then covered with sterile towels in such a way as to leave only the operation site exposed (Fig. 7). For extraoral procedures the mouth is also covered.

In the out-patient surgery the patient should be asked to wash the mouth thoroughly with a mouth wash and in the case of female patients all cosmetics should be removed. A sterile towel may then be pinned round the patient's neck and a sterile cap placed over the hair, to prevent contamination of the instruments or of the operator's hands (Fig.8). The patient's eyes are protected from the light and instruments by dark glasses.

The operation

All members of the team must work in a comfortable position to avoid fatigue. Modern equipment makes it possible for the surgeon and the assistant to work seated, which is much less tiring. With this in view the position and height of the table and chair, instrument trolleys and other apparatus are adjusted before the operation is commenced. In the dental surgery this should be done before the surgeon and his assistant scrub up.

The mouth can be held open with a rubber prop placed between the molar teeth. For operations under local anaesthesia a prop so used often helps the patient by resting his muscles and joints. Under general anaesthesia the mouth must not be opened by force because of the danger of fracturing teeth or damaging the temporomandibular joint. Pressure intraorally on the mental protuberance will open the mouth or gags may be gently applied to the teeth to separate the jaws.

Fig. 8 Patient prepared for out-patient surgery. Note protective eyewear.

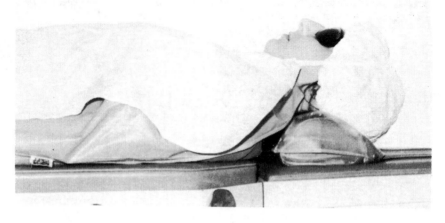

Before starting the operation the surgeon *must make sure he has the right patient and notes.* He then examines the mouth and radiographs to confirm the proposed operation. Where the patient is given a general anaesthetic teeth can be damaged or dislodged during induction. Especial care must be taken by anaesthetists and surgeons where loose teeth are present.

The close of the operation

The surgeon refers to the notes to confirm that all the surgery planned has been completed and tells the anaesthetist he is about to finish. He makes certain that all bleeding is controlled and that wound closure is satisfactory. He checks that packs or drains to be left in the mouth or wound are securely sutured in place. The mouth is searched for any clot, debris or swabs and a count is made of the teeth extracted, of swabs, needles and small instruments. With the anaesthetist's agreement the end of the throat pack may be drawn forward and any debris in the superficial layers removed from the mouth, after which the patient is handed over to the anaesthetist.

The surgeon will then write up the notes of the operation. This is done immediately for the information of the ward sister and whosoever should be called in an emergency.

Operation notes may be written in the following form:

Date	Name and number of theatre or surgery	Time of commencement of operation

Surgeon named.

Anaesthetist named.

1. Anaesthetic, Local anaesthetic, general anaesthetic, type, pack used.

2. Operation described logically. Incision – reflection – bone removed – teeth extracted or fracture reduced and fixed, etc. debridement of wound – closure of wound – sutures – dressings applied – removal of throat pack – condition of patients on finishing – time of completion of operation.

The assistant will remain with the anaesthetist to man the suction apparatus and to advise about the operation site. The patient must remain under the supervision of the anaesthetist preferably in a special recovery area, until he is sufficiently recovered to control his own airway.

It is usual in hospital practice for a nurse from the ward to fetch the patient from the operating theatre. The anaesthetist and the surgeon should tell her what procedures have taken place and give instructions verbally and in writing for the immediate post-operative nursing. She should be shown the site of the operation, the tongue suture if used, and any areas to be protected from pressure. Where intermaxillary fixation with wires or elastics is in place the nurse is shown which to cut to release the jaw in an emergency and given wire cutters for this purpose.

The patient will travel on a trolley equipped with an oxygen cylinder and mask, a tray containing tongue forceps, a gag and swabs firmly held in forceps. He will lie in his side in the tonsillar position to allow saliva or blood to drain from his mouth and will be accompanied back to the ward by two persons. One of these should be a trained nurse who gives the patient her undivided attention and in an emergency can send her companion for assistance.

Further reading

British Dental Association (1988) *Guide to blood-borne viruses and the control of cross-infection in dentistry.*

Joint Memoranda of The Medical Defence Union and the Royal College of Nursing (1978), *Safeguards against wrong operations* and *Safeguards against failure to remove swabs and instruments from patients.*

Medical Research Council (1968), 'Aseptic methods in the operating suite', *Lancet*, **1**, 705.

VII   Surgical principles and technique

The practice of surgery rests on certain fundamental principles which remain unchanged, though to apply them the surgeon may have to modify his technique to suit the anatomical field, the type of operation and the conditions obtaining at the time. The surgeon must have a clear and comprehensive knowledge of surgical physiology, of the anatomy of the region he is operating, and of the pathology of the condition under treatment.

Principle of painless surgery

Today it is accepted that all surgery should be painless. This is important to avoid psychological and physical stress to the patient which may predispose to shock, delay recovery and make surgery under local anaesthesia more difficult for the surgeon. In oral surgery it is wise for general anaesthetics to be administered by a specialist in this field, whereas the dental surgeon is usually highly skilled in giving his own local anaesthetic injections.

It is outside the scope of this book to discuss the administration of local and general anaesthetics. The choice between these will depend on surgical as well as medical considerations, and where doubt exists the decision should be made jointly with the anaesthetist. The dental surgeon may often have to guide the patient and the anaesthetist as to which is better.

The indications for general anaesthesia are: first, when there is an acute or subacute infection because an injection into the affected area may cause an exacerbation; second, where the operation involves several quadrants of the mouth, is lengthy, difficult, or of an alarming nature; third, for young children and nervous patients. General anaesthetics without intubation should not be used for procedures expected to last more than five minutes. Day-case surgery, where the patient is intubated and the post-operative period supervised by the nursing staff, is suitable for operations which can be completed within forty-five minutes.

Local anaesthesia is suitable for many minor oral surgical procedures. It is indicated where the patient has eaten recently and does not wish to wait and in certain medical conditions (such as chronic bronchitis). The combination of local anaesthesia and sedation, such as intravenous diazepam, is useful for the nervous patient. This technique requires well trained staff and adequate recovery facilities.

Principle of asepsis

Asepsis is the exclusion of micro-organisms from the operative field to prevent them entering the wound. The patient's mouth, however, cannot be sterilised and remains a source of infection. A pre-operative scaling, and good oral hygiene practised before operation will reduce the chance of gross contamination; moreover patients seem to acquire a degree of immunity to their own oral flora.

The sterile instruments, fluids and dressings used in oral surgery are laid up on a trolley. Where pre-packed instruments are not used this must be done with sterile forceps. The surgeon and assistant should wear sterile disposable gloves and only those instruments laid on the trolley should be handled. A third person should be present to adjust the operating lights and position of the patient.

Principle of minimal damage

Inexperienced surgeons often pay too much attention to the tooth, cyst, or tumour to be removed and too little to the tissues left after surgery is complete. Certain radical operations may regrettably require the sacrifice of vital structures but this does not often apply in oral surgery, and damage or loss of function as a result of carelessness or lack of foresight is inexcusable.

The commonest causes of trauma are poorly planned operations with ill-designed flaps, a careless approach to bone removal and tooth extraction, and excessive use of force by the surgeon or his assistant in dissection, retraction of flaps and in the use of elevators, burs and chisels. These practices increase post-operative pain and swelling and delay healing. They not only interfere with healing but increase the possibility of infection because they leave behind pieces of dead bone, tooth and mutilated soft tissues.

Principle of adequate access

Incision and flap

Access to the site of operation is gained by cutting the skin or mucous membrane and by dissecting through this incision to lay back a flap. The site, size and form of the incision is planned to give the best possible approach with the least danger to important nearby structures. The operation completed, the flap has a second and equally important function, that of providing the first dressing to the wound. To do this it must be large enough to give easy access, be mobilised with sufficient subcutaneous tissue to give adequate support and bring with it a good blood supply. It should have healthy, clean edges which will heal by first intention. This means that, in the mouth, when the mucoperiosteum is reflected the mucosa and periosteum must not be separated. The incision must be so designed that it does not cut across the blood supply to the flap but includes the vessels that supply that area of skin or mucous membrane, otherwise the edges may slough and healing is delayed (Fig. 9).

Fig. 9 (a) *Above:* Correct design of the buccal flap to ensure a satisfactory blood supply to all parts. *Below:* Cross-section of satisfactory incision made with the scalpel blade vertical to the surface of the skin. (b) *Above:* Incorrect design of buccal flap. *Below:* Cross-section of an incision made with the scalpel blade held obliquely.

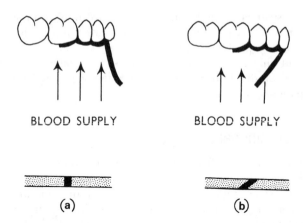

Where it covers a cavity in bone, it should be of such a size that when replaced the line of the incision rests securely on bone.

Incision. The scalpel is held in a pen-grip and the hand is supported against slipping. The incision is made with one firm, slow stroke of a sharp blade which is kept vertical to the epithelial surface. The bow is used for cutting, the point being kept above the skin or mucous membrane as a guide to the depth at which the incision is being made. (Fig. 10).

The point is used at the beginning and end of the incision to ensure an even depth of cut along the whole length. Mucoperiosteum should be cut through its full thickness down on to bone at *one* stroke.

Dissection. The mucoperiosteal flap may be reflected with a Howarth's raspatory used as a periosteal elevator. This is first inserted into the incision and, starting in the buccal sulcus where the periosteum is loosely attached, the first few millimetres at the edge of the flap are gently freed along its periphery. Thereafter, it is reflected, evenly along its whole length by a clean movement with the end of the Howarth's raspatory pressed and kept firmly against the bone. Lifting movements are to be avoided as they tend to tear the tissues.

A skin flap is raised by separating it, with sufficient supporting tissue, from the underlying structures either by blunt dissection, using scissors, or, where necessary, by cutting with a scalpel. The essential point is to maintain an even depth of supporting tissue with an adequate blood supply and to avoid 'buttonholing' the flap. The deeper tissues are explored by blunt dissection with either sinus forceps, the fingers, or where delicate structures are involved by separating each layer by gently packing wet gauze between

Fig. 10 The scalpel held in the pen-grip and the bow of a No. 15 blade used to make the incision. Note the fingers supported on the teeth.

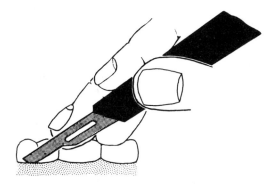

them. Connective tissue, muscle, and bone must be identified, laid open in turn, and all important structures carefully preserved.

Cutting of bone

In oral surgery the cutting of bone to give access is done with burs, chisels, gouges, rongeurs and files. Ideally the operator should master the use of all these.

Burs. Dental burs of medium size, either rosehead (Ash 7-16) or fissure (Ash 7-12), are used. Satisfactory cutting with fine control can only be attained using high speeds and minimal pressure. To avoid overheating of the tissues and clogging of the bur this must be irrigated with sterile saline.

Burs can be used in two ways, either to grind bone away or to remove blocks of bone. Grinding is done with rosehead or fissure burs preferably used with a gentle sweeping movement over the whole length of the area concerned, thereby leaving a smooth even edge. Blocks of bone are removed using fissure burs (Ash size 7) to make cuts through the cortex into the medulla round an area which can then be prised out.

Chisels. These may be used to great advantage in young patients, under forty years of age, where the natural lines of cleavage along the 'grain' of the bone are present. In the mandible these run vertically in the ascending ramus (almost parallel to the posterior border) and horizontally in the body (parallel to the occlusal surface). In the maxilla there is no true grain, but the thin plates of bone are easily cut. In older patients (over forty years) the use of chisels is contraindicated as the bone is brittle and the mandible may shatter in unpredictable planes. With sharp chisels and carefully placed stopcuts the degree of control exercised is not inferior to that obtained with burs. Chisels may be used either by hand or more usually with a mallet. In either case they must be supported firmly against slipping. Some resilience should be provided in the mallet either in the handle or by use of a soft head.

The chisel may be used to plane bone away or to cut out blocks of bone. The direction in which the chisel cuts is determined by the angle of the bevelled surface. When used as a plane the bevelled face is placed against the bone and driven along at the required depth to shave off successive wafers. To remove blocks of bone the bevelled surface is usually turned towards the bone which is to be left (Fig. 11).

The angle at which the chisel is held is determined by the amount of chamfer which the surgeon wishes to leave on this bone edge. It is wise to outline the area with shallow cuts made with a small (3 mm) chisel before applying a broader (5 mm) blade; this prevents splitting along the grain over a long distance.

Chisels and burs. These may be combined by using a rosehead bur (No. 7) to drill holes to the required depth at intervals of 3–5 mm along the planned line of the cut. The holes are then joined with a chisel and the cut deepened gradually till the bone splits off. This method is especially useful for removing large pieces of bone safely.

Rongeurs and files. These instruments are used mostly for trimming and smoothing bone edges when the operation has been completed. The rongeurs may also be used for cutting alveolar bone in alveolectomy and thin plates of bone such as those covering dental cysts.

Retraction °

Retraction has two objects, to provide free access for the surgeon and to protect the tissues. It is the most important task undertaken by the assistant, which, if badly performed, can be a positive hindrance. The tissue layers divided by the incision and the dissection are gently held back with instruments (Fig. 12). There should be no tugging or rough handling, for if this is necessary the incision is too small and needs to be enlarged. Retractors must not be moved without warning as they may accidentally obscure the

Fig. 11 (a) Upper chisel being used as a plane with the bevel towards the bone. Lower chisel being used to remove a block of bone with bevel turned towards the bone to be retained. (b) Note the bevel produced on the bone when the chisel is correctly used.

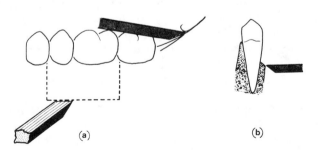

(a)   (b)

Fig. 12 Retractors, from left to right, are Ward's gum retractor with a broad blade where it retracts the cheek, Bowdler Henry rake retractor for muco-periosteal flaps, and Lack's tongue retractor.

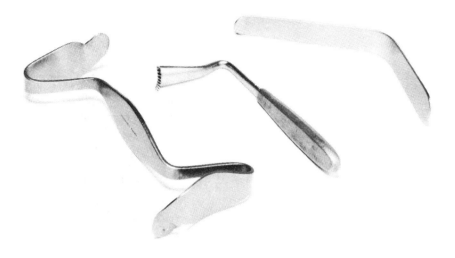

field or deflect an instrument. To keep still for periods, without tiring, the hands must be in a comfortable position, if possible supported in some way. Thus the blade of the retractor under a mucoperiosteal flap should rest against the alveolar bone. The surgeon should pause at intervals to allow his assistant to rest and readjust his position.

Damage may also occur from compressing or cutting the lips or cheeks against the teeth. To avoid undue pressure at any one point, the lips, tongue and cheeks are best held back by broad-bladed instruments. Unfortunately, this is more often done by the handles of retractors, the blades of which are holding back flaps in the mouth and only a few of which are designed for both purposes. Sutures of thick silk can be passed through all these structures, and through mucoperiosteal flaps, to hold them. The tongue can conveniently be drawn laterally by the use of a teaspoon with the handle suitably bent for attaching it to a mouthprop (Fig. 13).

Cleansing the field of operation

The assistant cleanses the field of operation of fluids and loose debris, which might obscure the surgeon's view or remain in the wound to become foreign bodies. Large fragments should be lifted out with fine forceps as soon as they are seen, otherwise they may be lost. Blood, water, and the minute debris from cutting hard tissues with the dental bur can be removed by suction. The tip of the sucker should be kept in one position, preferably at the point of dependent drainage, as moving it continually can interfere

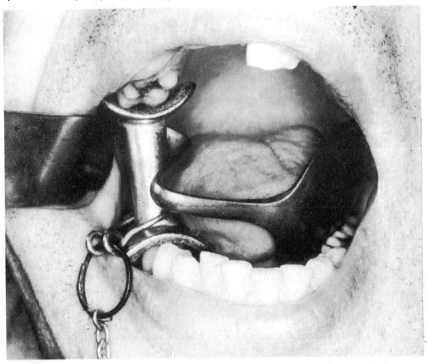

with the surgeon's instrumentation and, if rapid, causes a visual kaleidoscope effect. At intervals sterile water must be aspirated to prevent blood clotting in the tubing or connections. Large particles of bone or tags of tissue are avoided; they are sometimes musical but will eventually block the tubing. As this occurs not infrequently, a spare 'head' together with a stilette is needed. The sucker should not be used as a retractor or to explore wounds or sockets as it can cause damage and may encourage bleeding. The use of swabs in similar circumstances avoids this.

Principle of arrest of haemorrhage

The natural arrest of haemorrhage and the pathological conditions which may lead to abnormal bleeding together with their management have been discussed in Chapter III. At operation the arrest of primary haemorrhage depends on the application of pressure to the vessel walls which to be effective must be maintained for at least the time taken for the blood to clot. Haemostatis must be achieved in each quadrant of the mouth before continuing to other procedures in a new area. Reactionary and secondary haemorrhage are discussed in Chapter X.

Soft tissues

Digital pressure. This is particularly useful for capillary or venous bleeding and as an immediate measure when a large vessel has been cut. It is applied either by compressing the tissues, or the offending vessel, against bone or in certain situations, such as the lip, by exerting pressure between index finger and thumb. The lingual artery may be controlled by drawing the tongue forward so that the artery is pressed against the hyoid bone. The facial artery crosses the lower border of the mandible where digital pressure may be applied.

Haemostats or artery forceps. Where a vessel is cut during operation it must be found swiftly and secured with artery forceps. For small vessels the haemostats may be removed after twisting two or three times, but on larger vessels they must be replaced by ligatures.

Ligatures. Direct ligature of a vessel is performed preferably before division. Artery forceps are placed above and below where the cut is to be made and after division resorbable ligatures are firmly tied and the haemostats removed (Fig. 14).

In major haemorrhage from the jaws not controlled by local measures it is on occasion necessary to ligate the external carotid artery. The collateral blood supply and anastomosis is so good in the face that it is often necessary to do this on both sides, if it is to be effective. A sufficient blood supply is still maintained by the other lesser vessels serving this area.

Packing. As a temporary measure ribbon gauze soaked in saline may be packed into operative or traumatic wounds and held under pressure for a short interval to arrest haemorrhage.

Posture. The position of the patient both during and after operation may help to reduce the blood pressure in the bleeding part. In dental haemorrhage the patient is kept sitting upright or propped up with pillows in bed unless shocked or fainting.

Electrocoagulation. This may be applied directly to the vessels or by passing the current through the artery forceps clamping the vessels. The anaesthetist should be warned that electrocoagulation is to be used in case explosive anaesthetic gases are being employed.

Fig. 14 Use of haemostats. Note the position of the lower haemostats on the vessel so that after division the beaks curve upwards out of the would (as on the upper haemostats) to facilitate passing and tying of the ligature.

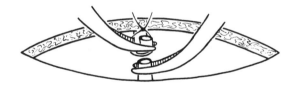

Capillary oozing from bone surfaces may be controlled by burnishing the bone with a small instrument or by applying for a few minutes hot packs prepared by soaking gauze squares in very hot water and wringing out the excess. Horsley's bone wax rubbed into the surface of the bone is also very effective in occluding small vessels.

Where an artery is bleeding from a bone surface it may be compressed by driving a chisel into the bone near to it and forcing a wedge of bone against the vessel.

Principle of debridement (toilet of wounds)

The operation completed, the wound is prepared for closure by careful cleansing to remove debris, a major cause of post-operative infection. Pathological tissue, such as tooth follicle or sinus tracts is excised. The bone cavity is saucerized where necessary, and the edges filed to a clean smooth finish without sharp projections. The flaps are trimmed of all necrotic tissue or tags. Tooth chips and loose pieces of bone, not attached to periosteum, are removed from the wound which is then thoroughly irrigated with saline.

Principle of drainage

Wounds need to drain freely after operation where they are contaminated or infected, where an abscess has been incised, or where immediate closure is made over a dead space which may fill with blood or serum and subsequently become infected.

Fine superficial drains. These are made of pieces of rubber glove and are used in wounds of the face to allow escape of tissue exudate. They are usually removed after forty eight-hours (Fig. 15a).

Fig. 15 Drains: (a) rubber glove drain: (b) corrugated drain; (c) tube drain with holes. Note that all these are held in place with sutures.

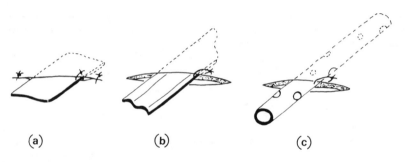

(a)   (b)   (c)

Larger superficial drains. Corrugated rubber or a Yeates drain is used in a dental abscess to keep the wound edges apart and allow thick pus to flow freely (Fig. 15b). Though chiefly used for extraoral incisions and drainage they are necessary for large collections of pus drained intraorally.

Deep drains. Tubing, sometimes with small holes cut in its walls, is used in osteomyelitis of the jaws or to drain the antrum through the nose. The tubes must be of sufficient diameter to ensure the free passage of fluid and to allow irrigation with saline or antibiotic solutions (Fig. 15c).

Vacuum drains. These are inserted at a point remote from the wound by means of a central sharp stylet. The stylet is then withdrawn leaving the tube drain in position. The latter is attached to a plastic bottle from which the air has been expressed. The advantages of vacuum drains are that they are inserted away from the operation wound and that the negative pressure developed assists removal of fluid.

Drains should be inserted into a cavity at its most dependent point and they must be fixed by a suture or some other device to prevent them falling out of, or being drawn into, the wound. They should be examined daily to ensure that they are patent and serving their function. They are removed when the discharge has ceased, usually between the third and seventh day. Long drains may be shortened before this, particularly when they are near major vessels which they may erode.

An entry must be made in the patient's records both when they are put in and when they are removed.

Principle of repair of wounds

Before commencing closure the surgeon makes sure that the operation has been satisfactorily completed, that bleeding is arrested and that all swabs, instruments and teeth are accounted for. Closure is carried out by suturing the wound for which purpose many forms of needle holder, needle and suture material are available.

Needle holder. The Ward needle holder is designed for use in the mouth. It has long handles to reach to the back of this cavity and an eye in one of the beaks to allow the needle to be held and driven through the tissues in the long axis of the needle holder (Fig. 16).

Needles. These may be round or triangular in cross-section; the latter are called 'cutting needles'. They may be of various shapes but the half-round or curved needle is used on the mucous membranes and skin of the face. The size of the needle should be such that it can be passed through the flap without ever holding it by either the tail or the point, where it may easily be broken.

Suture materials Those in common use are nylon, silk, catgut and polyglycolic acid. Twisted silk is the softest and is to be preferred for mucous membranes and skin. Soluble catgut and polyglycolic acid which dissolve out at different

Fig. 16 Suturing kit showing, *left to right*, Ward's needle holder, toothed tissue forceps, suture scissors, and, *above*, suture.

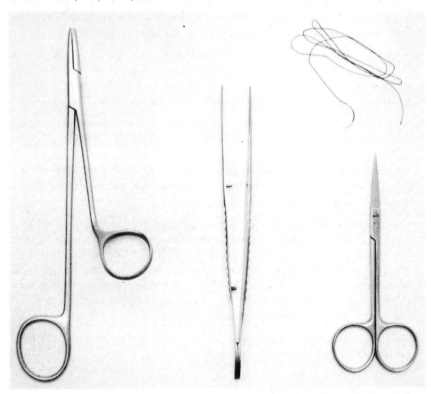

rates according to their mode of manufacture are used for suturing connective tissues and muscle. They may be used for young children or the mentally subnormal where difficulty in removal is anticipated. Silk is made in various gauges from very small (0.1 metric or 10/0) to medium (3.5 metric or 0/0) or gross (8 metric to 6), fused to an eyeless needle by the manufacturers.

Suturing.   To suture the mucoperiosteum the edges of the wound are apposed to confirm that closure can be made without tension. Where one side is fixed to bone the first 3 mm of the margin are freed to make the passage of the needle easy. The flap is picked up and held everted with toothed tissue forceps applied at right angles to the free edge of the flap (Fig. 17). A curved cutting needle (22 mm.) with silk (gauge 2 metric or 3/0) is passed through from the outer surface of the mucoperiosteum close to the tissue forceps which splint the flap against the pressure from the needle. The suture must go through the periosteum and should be placed about 3 mm from the free edge to prevent it pulling out when tied. The other side is similarly everted and the needle passed through from the raw surface with an equal bite. To make sure that the final position will be satisfactory the

Fig. 17 (a), (b) and (c) show eversion of the flap and the needle passed obliquely through the tissue; (d) tying of the suture everts the edges of the wound; (e) removal of sutures, by cutting at A and thereby avoiding drawing the exposed part of the suture through the tissues.

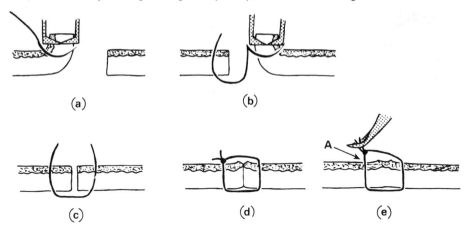

(a)   (b)

(c)   (d)   (e)

margins of the wound are drawn together with the suture before it is tied with a surgeon's knot (Fig. 18). It should not be tied too tightly as this may make the edges overlap and because subsequent swelling may cause ischaemia at the wound margins. Sufficient sutures are inserted to prevent the wound gaping at any point.

Skin incisions are closed in layers, the fascial and muscle planes being identified and re-apposed. They are sutured with catgut or polyglycolic acid, the knot of which should be tied inwards and the free ends cut very short to avoid irritation. The deep sutures should take all the necessary strain so that the skin lies in correct apposition and may be stitched without tension, which is a cause of scarring. It is very important that the skin margins are held everted with the raw surfaces in apposition to ensure rapid healing (Fig. 17).

Types of suture

Simple interrupted sutures. These are of almost universal application. They are inserted singly through each side of the wound and tied with a surgeon's knot (Fig. 18). Several of these may be used at short intervals between 4 and 8 mm apart to close large wounds, so that the tension is shared and therefore not high at any one point (Fig. 19a). When put in correctly they will evert the edges of the flap. Should one break or pull out only this one need be replaced. The wound is free of interference between each stitch and is easy to keep clean.

Horizontal mattress suture. This has the property of everting the mucosal or skin margins, thereby bringing greater areas of raw tissue into contact. For this reason it is useful for closing wounds over boney deficiencies such as oro-antral fistulae or cyst cavities (Fig. 19b).

Fig. 18 Surgeon's knot: (a) knot in detail; (b) first part of the knot made by passing suture round needle holder; (c) and (d) short free end grasped and knot slid off beaks; (e) and (f) second part of knot made by passing suture round the needle holder in the opposite direction.

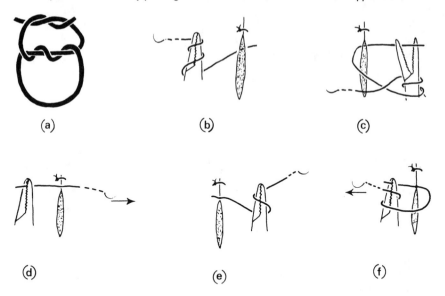

Vertical mattress sutures. Specially designed for use in the skin, they pass through it at two levels, one deep to provide support and adduction of the wound surface at a depth and one superficial to draw the edges together and evert them.

Continuous sutures. These all suffer from the great disadvantage that if they cut out at one point the suture slackens along the whole length of the wound which will then gape open. They have the advantage in the mouth that only two knots with their associated tags are present. The simple continuous suture (Fig. 19c), though easy to insert, applies its pull on the wound in an oblique direction. The continuous blanket stitch suture is far more stable and firm and gives traction on the wound edges at right angles to the wound (Fig. 19d). The purse-string suture is useful as a deep suture for wounds of the skin of the face, but care must be taken that in drawing the suture taut there is no wrinkling or creasing of the skin edges.

Knots. The knots used to tie sutures are the reef-knot and surgeon's knot. They may be tied with the fingers but this is difficult to do in the mouth and it is important to master the technique of tying them with the needle holder as illustrated (Fig. 18). The knot when tied must lie well on one side of the line of the wound.

Removal of sutures. Sutures in mucous membrane are removed after five to seven days. In the skin alternative stitches are often taken out about the third to fifth day and the remainder between the fifth and eighth days. A good guide is that as soon as they begin to get loose they should be taken out. They should first be cleaned and then removed as shown in Fig. 17.

Fig. 19 Sutures: (a) simple interrupted; (b) horizontal mattress; (c) simple continuous; (d) continuous blanket stitch.

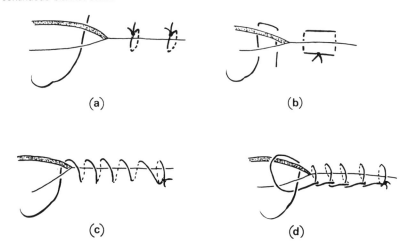

(a)

(b)

(c)

(d)

Principle of control and prevention of infection of wounds

The incidence of post-operative infection will be reduced by careful pre-operative preparation, an aseptic technique, minimal trauma and adequate drainage. Post-operatively the tissues may be protected by the use of dressings.

In the mouth surgical incisions are not dressed except where there is a deficiency of mucous membrane over bone, when packs are used to cover it. Small skin incisions are normally dressed with dry gauze, until the formation of serous exudate has stopped when they are best left uncovered. More extensive wounds and abrasions may be covered with tulle-gras and dry gauze strapped into position with adhesive surgical tape. Where a drain is *in situ*, gauze is placed round it for support, and to absorb the discharge cotton wool is held over it by a bandage or strapping which should completely cover the dressing.

Packs are used to protect exposed bone or to prevent skin or mucous membrane from closing over a wound which should heal from its base by granulation. They can in no way serve as drains. Ribbon gauze impregnated with B.I.P.P., or Whitehead's varnish is packed firmly but not tightly into the cavity. When inserted under a general anaesthetic, packs must be sutured into place lest they come loose and obstruct the airway. They should not be changed too frequently and *both insertion and removal must be entered in the patient's notes*.

Antibacterial therapy. Views on the prophylactic use of antibiotics vary but on no account should they take the place of an aseptic technique. In oral surgery it is impossible to obtain a sterile field and many patients present with acute or chronic inflammatory conditions such as advanced periodontal disease, pericoronitis, or contaminated fratures. For this reason many oral surgeons prefer to operate under an antibiotic cover, but it should not be prescribed routinely. Each case must be assessed individually and bacterial culture and antibiotic sensitivity tests obtained wherever possible. The prescription of antibacterial drugs is discussed in Chapter V.

Principle of support of the patient

The pre- and post-operative care and the general support of the patient have been discussed in Chapter II.

Further reading

Kirk, R. M. (1989), *Basic Surgical Techniques*, 3rd edn. Churchill Livingstone, Edinburgh.

VIII Extraction of teeth and roots

The indications for the extraction of teeth are well known and include caries, acute infections, periodontal disease, trauma and orthodontic reasons.

Examination and assessment

A full medical history is necessary before attempting extractions as these are contraindicated in certain conditions such as leukaemias and for patients whose jaws have undergone irradiation. Other medical conditions which need special preparation such as bone dysplasias, cardiac and haemorrhagic diseases are discussed in Chapter III. Any previous difficulty with extractions including post-operative bleeding or infection is noted and if serious in extent investigated further.

Clinical examination. The patient's sex, age, general build and bone structure are significant. Heavily built men, particularly Negroes, have teeth difficult to extract whilst in old age roots are brittle and the bone sclerosed, the so-called 'glass in concrete syndrome'. Access may be difficult in children who have small mouths and in patients with facial scars or trismus.

The tooth to be extracted is examined. Teeth misplaced palatally or lingually, rotated, inclined, or single standing teeth in occlusion, are all potentially difficult. Certain teeth frequently have abnormal root formation, particularly the upper and lower third molars. Heavily filled and dead teeth or those suffering from long-standing periodontal disease tend to become brittle. Periodontal disease predisposes to post-operative bleeding and infection. In acute ulcerative gingivitis or where the gingival condition suggests a blood dyscrasia all extractions must be delayed until these have been treated.

Radiographic examination. The nature of the root form and bone structure can only be determined from radiographs, and ideally these should always be taken before extraction, but in practice this is done when the history or examination suggest the extractions will be difficult. It should be a routine procedure for all lower third molars and misplaced teeth. Intraoral periapical views should show the whole of the crown, root and alveolus and demonstrate the relationship of the roots to such important structures as the maxillary sinus and the inferior dental canal. Radiographs must be examined carefully as certain features, such as extra roots on molar teeth, are easily missed.

Assessment. All the findings on examination and radiography are considered, particularly the number, size, shape and position of roots and any signs of hypercementosis or resorption. The condition of the supporting bone, especially evidence of sclerosis, resorption or of secondary conditions such as apical granulomas and cysts, is noted. Where any of these complications occur the treatment plan should be modified to meet them.

Extraction of teeth

Forceps

These have two blades with sharp edges to cut the periodontal fibres. The blades are wedge-shaped to dilate the socket and are hollowed on their inner surface to fit the roots. They are made in various sizes and a range should be available so that a pair may be selected which fit snugly round the roots and have even contact with the cementum over a wide area. One- or two-point contact is bad and prevents the tooth being gripped firmly. They should engage only the roots and never the crowns of the teeth.

The blades are hinged which allows them to close and grasp the root. The handles act as a lever which gives the operator a mechanical advantage. The farther from the blades the surgeon grasps the handles the less effort he will have to make to apply force to the tooth. In order to drive the forceps blade straight up the long axis of the tooth the shape of the handle is varied. Lower forceps have handles at right angles to the blades, upper forceps are straight for anterior teeth and cranked for the posteriors. For the upper third molars the beaks as well as the handles are bent (Fig. 20).

Certain forceps ('full forceps') have specially designed blades to fit the molar teeth. They do not penetrate up the periodontal membrane but grip the tooth at the bifurcation and by moving the roots dilate the socket. They have an application where penetration is difficult and the bone is resilient. This applies to young people under twenty whose periodontal condition is good, roots are not brittle and bone not sclerosed.

Extraction of teeth with forceps

The extraction of teeth is a surgical operation based primarily on an anatomical appreciation of their attachment in the jaws. First the soft tissues of the gingival attachment and periodontal membrane are cut to separate the tooth from bone. Next the socket is dilated either by instruments with wedge-shaped blades which are driven along the periodontal membrane, or by moving the root to expand its bony socket. Finally when the tooth is loose it may be drawn out of the alveolus. When completed with forceps, extractions are performed in two movements.

First movement. This is the same for all the teeth of both jaws. The forceps are applied on the buccal and the palatal or lingual aspect of the tooth, regardless of whether it is normally or abnormally positioned in the arch. For multirooted teeth, unless full forceps are used, the blades must be kept on a root, not the bifurcation. The blades are passed carefully under the gingival margin of the tooth avoiding damage to the soft tissues, and driven up or down the roots (according to the jaw concerned) in the same plane

Fig. 20 Forceps. *Left to right:* Upper straight forceps; upper premolar and molar forceps; upper bayonets and lower root forceps; and side views of the upper straight, premolar and bayonet forceps.

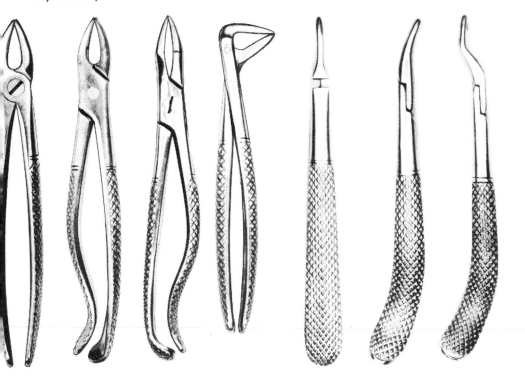

as the long axis of the tooth to penetrate as far as possible. This can only be done successfully if the forceps blades are held sufficiently apart that they do *not* grip the tooth root.

Considerable force is used, particularly in the upper jaw. In the lower jaw this must be limited to that which the operator can counteract by supporting the mandible with his free hand. Whilst driving up the root in this way the blades should be in contact with the root surface but not gripping it. This movement cuts the gingival attachment and periodontal membrane and also uses the wedge-shaped blades to dilate the socket. Conical roots may sometimes be extracted by this movement alone.

Second movement. The first movement completed, the blades of the forceps are closed to grasp the root and a second movement is performed which by moving the tooth roots uses them to dilate further the socket and to free them from the periodontal membrane. During this action, to prevent the blades slipping off the tooth, a firm vertical pressure up or down the long axis of the root must be maintained. The character of the second movement depends on two factors. Firstly, in both upper and lower jaws the palatal or lingual alveolar bone is thicker than the buccal bone, and secondly, the

Fig. 21 *Left:* Method of holding upper forceps. Note grip and position of the blades on root, *not* crown. *Right:* Method of holding lower forceps.

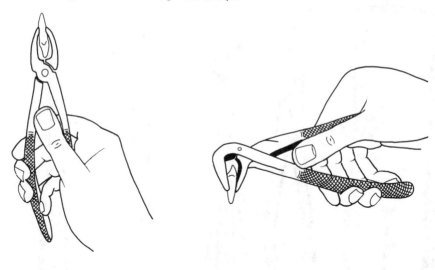

anatomy of the roots of the various classes of teeth differs both in their number and shape.

The use of excess force is avoided, and every effort is made to develop 'feeling' through the forceps. This enables the surgeon to recognise resistance to excursions in certain directions and to exploit other movements which the tooth will follow more easily, and so to extract always along the line of least resistance.

Upper incisors and canines. These have single, conical roots and are therefore rotated with a purposeful action, the forceps turning through as wide an arc as possible without damaging adjacent teeth (Fig. 22). The upper

Fig. 22 Movements in the extraction of teeth: (a) rotation; (b) buccal outward movement.

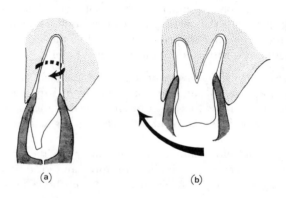

(a)   (b)

canine, because its root is slightly flattened mesiodistally, can be extracted by an outward buccal movement if it is resistant to rotation.

Upper premolars. These have either one strong root markedly flattened mediodistally or two fine conical roots placed buccally and palatally. They are extracted by a limited bucco-palatal movement lest the apices should break.

Upper first and second molars. Both these teeth have three roots which are usually somewhat flattened. The palatal diverges strongly from the two buccal roots. They are taken bucally with a long, steady movement whilst the upward pressure is maintained (Fig. 22). Palatal movement is contra-indicated as it may cause the palatal root to fracture.

Upper third molars. The morphology of these roots varies widely; some are fused, others have three fine roots. They are extracted in the same way as the other upper molars, but it is wise to take a radiograph first.

Lower incisors and canines. The roots of these teeth are flattened mesiodistally and as the buccal plate of bone is very weak they are extracted with an outward buccal movement.

Lower premolars. These have conical roots and are therefore rotated.

Lower first and second molars. Their roots are flattened mesiodistally. They should be extracted by a buccal movement while the downward pressure is maintained.

Lower third molars. A wide variation occurs in their root form and in their position in the mandible as they are often misplaced or inclined. Radiographs should always be taken before extraction which may require an open or transalveolar approach.

Deciduous teeth. The upper and lower incisors and canines are extracted with the same movements used for their permanent successors. The molar teeth, however, have divergent roots which enclose the follicle of the developing premolar teeth and it is possible to remove or damage the latter when extracting a deciduous molar. Great care must be taken in using the forceps, which should not be driven too far up the periodontal membrane. They are applied to the tooth *root*, avoiding the bifurcation under which the permanent tooth germ nestles (Fig. 23).

Where, owing to caries or a fracture of the tooth during surgery, a deciduous molar root is retained which cannot be grasped with the forceps, it may be extracted by applying a right-angled Warwick James's elevator to the mesial aspect of mesial roots or distal aspect of distal roots to elevate them gently along their natural curvature. Should there be a risk of damaging the underlying permanent tooth, then the retained root is best left and the patient's parent told the reason.

Difficult extractions. The ultimate aim of the student is to acquire the ability to assess the tooth he wishes to extract and to modify his technique accordingly. During the operation the second movement is always slow,

Fig. 23 Position of forceps on deciduous molars: *left*, incorrect, *right*, correct position of blade on the deciduous root.

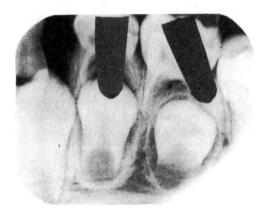

steady and purposeful and not a series of short, jerky, shaking gestures which are both ineffective and unpleasant for the patient.

Should there be complete resistance to the forceps when the usual pressure is applied the operation is stopped and a new assessment made with radiographs. Where necessary the roots are freed through a transalveolar approach by making a flap, removing bone and dividing the tooth, rather than by exerting more and more force till the tooth breaks.

Elevators

Elevators are single-bladed instruments for extracting teeth and roots, which they do by moving them out of the sockets along a path determined by the natural curvature of the roots. They are applied to the cementum on any surface, usually the mesial, distal or buccal, at a point (the point of application) where there is alveolar bone to provide them with a fulcrum. An adjoining tooth must never be used as the fulcrum, unless it is also to be extracted at the same visit, as it might be loosened accidentally.

Elevators are supported against slipping by resting the forefingers of the working hand on an adjacent tooth or the jaw (Fig. 24). They may be pushed firmly *between tooth and bone* to engage the point of application, but when elevating the tooth the force used is carefully controlled and should not exceed that which can be applied by rotating the instrument between finger and thumb (Fig. 25). Where this is insufficient to move the tooth, other measures such as removal of bone or division of the tooth may be necessary. An elevator should never be used as a Class 1 lever, that is like a crowbar, as bone will be crushed and the mechanical advantage is such that the jaw may be fractured.

Throughout elevation its effects on the tooth to be extracted and on the adjacent teeth is carefully watched so that ineffective or damaging

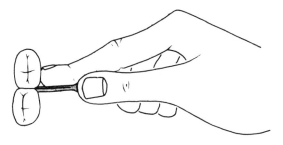

movements are avoided. Where a tooth is standing distal to the one to be extracted every precaution must be taken not to transmit injurious forces to it.

Many elevators have been designed to exert more than finger and thumb pressure, but these should not be used to extract teeth. A description follows of some elevators which are safe to use, provided the above principles are obeyed.

Coupland's elevator.   This is made in three sizes; each has a single blade not unlike that of the forceps (Fig. 26). It may be used as a wedge to dilate the socket when driven vertically up the periodontal membrane. More commonly it is used as a pulley lever, the mechanical advantage being obtained through the greater diameter of the handle over that of the blade (Fig. 25). When inserted horizontally between tooth and bone the sharp blade engages the point of application on the cementum and, with the alveolar bone as a fulcrum, the handle is rotated to lift the root out of its socket along its line of withdrawal (Figs. 24 and 25).

Fig. 25 (a) *Left:* Correct point of application between tooth and bone. *Right:* Incorrect application between tooth and tooth. (b) The force applied at the elevator handle (*E*) is multiplied by the ratio of the diameter of the handle (*D*) to the diameter of the blade (*d*) at the point of application.

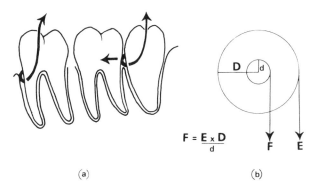

$$F = \frac{E \times D}{d}$$

(a)   (b)

Fig. 26 Elevators. *Left to right:* Coupland's elevators 1, 2, 3; Cryer's elevators, left and right; Warwick James elevators, left and right.

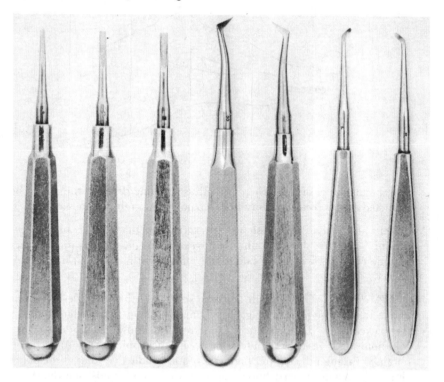

Warwick James elevators. These are a pair of fine elevators (Fig. 26). The blade may be driven into the periodontal membrane to engage the root either mesially, distally or buccally and the handle rotated to lift it from its socket. A straight Warwick James elevator is also available and used in a similar way to the Coupland's elevator.

Cryer's elevators. These are made in pairs, a right and left, and have a short, sharp-pointed, triangular blade at right angles to the handle (Fig. 26). They are used exactly like the right-angled Warwick James elevators but the larger, stronger blade gives them a superior mechanical advantage particularly when they are applied bucally to roots or to molar teeth at their bifurcation.

In molar teeth, especially in the mandible, where one root is retained a Cryer's elevator may be inserted into the adjacent empty socket and the sharp point used to remove the inter-radicular bone until it can engage the cementum. The bone is flaked away starting at the occlusal margin of the septum and working down towards the root apex.

The combined use of forceps and elevators. The combined use of these instruments will enable the operator to exploit the best qualities of both and thereby develop a gentle progressive technique. The first instrument to be applied should be a Coupland's elevator driven vertically up the long axis. This will cut the periodontal membrane and dilate the bony socket on both buccal and lingual aspects and indicate if undue resistance is present. As soon as there is some response to the elevators forceps may be applied.

The supporting hand

The responsibility for seeing that the jaws are adequately supported rests with the operator, and his free hand is used for this purpose. This is particularly important in the mandible where the downward force must be resisted. Under local anaesthesia, a prop may be inserted and the patient can help by biting firmly on this. Under general anaesthesia in the dental chair the anaesthetist assists by supporting the mandible at the angles. Satisfactory support is equally important when using forceps or elevators (Fig. 27).

The other function of the supporting hand is to retract the cheeks and tongue and to protect the tissues. This is done by placing a finger and thumb (or two fingers) one on each side of the gum on the buccal and the lingual or palatal aspects of the tooth. At the same time the operator is able to feel that the blades of the forceps are indeed under the mucous membrane and correctly applied to the tooth. During the second movement of extraction, the watching fingers can feel any slipping of the forceps on the tooth or any tendency of adjacent teeth to move, or alveolar bone to fracture. When working on the maxilla the free fingers of the supporting hand should be kept closed to avoid the fingers causing accidental damage to the patient's eyes.

Stance

The right-handed operator stands facing the patient to the left of the chair but not too close as this makes lighting difficult. The stance has been compared to that of a boxer about to deliver a blow. The left foot is advanced, the weight balanced on both feet, with the arms slightly bent. The left hand is put forward to support the jaw whilst the right grasps the forceps. This position is adopted for the extraction of all upper teeth and for those in the left mandible (Fig. 28).

Teeth in the right mandible are extracted from behind the patient. The feet are apart with the right slightly advanced, and the left arm is placed round the patient's head to support the lower jaw (Figs. 27 and 28).

Chair position

The patient should be seated upright with the buttocks well back in the chair and the head supported with the neck slightly extended. The height of the chair is adjusted so that the occlusal plane of the teeth is level with the operator's shoulder when extracting from the upper jaw, and with his elbow when extracting from the lower jaw.

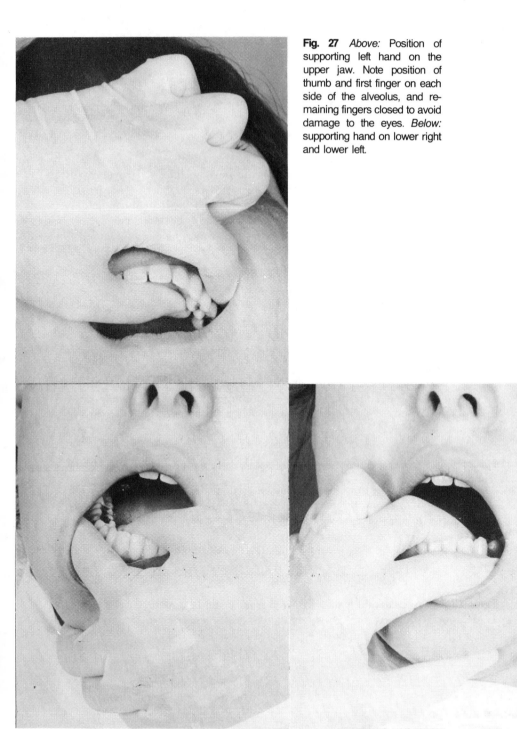

Fig. 27 *Above:* Position of supporting left hand on the upper jaw. Note position of thumb and first finger on each side of the alveolus, and remaining fingers closed to avoid damage to the eyes. *Below:* supporting hand on lower right and lower left.

Order of extraction of teeth

To prevent blood from the sockets of extracted teeth obscuring the field of operation it is usual to remove lower teeth before uppers, and posteriors before anteriors. Unnecessary movement to and fro about the chair is avoided by starting multiple extractions with those from the right mandible, which are the only ones done from behind on the sitting patient.

It is wise to begin with the most painful tooth when undertaking multiple extractions lest any surgical or anaesthetic difficulty prevents the completion of the operation. Similarly, when working under local anaesthesia only one quadrant of the mouth should be injected at a time. When the surgery in this area has been successfully completed a new quadrant may be injected. It is better to take out teeth from one side of the mouth only at one visit, thereby leaving the other comfortable for chewing.

The extraction of a great many teeth at one out-patient sitting is contraindicated as it may upset the patient and the blood loss can be considerable. It is not possible to state a figure for the number of teeth as much will depend on the surgical difficulty and the patient's health and morale, but between four and eight would seem reasonable. Where it is necessary to do more at one visit the patient should be kept in the recovery room for at least half an hour post-operatively and then accompanied home by a relative. Alternatively the patient should be admitted to hospital.

Extractions under general anaesthesia

The pre-operative preparation for general anaesthesia is discussed in Chapter II.

The surgeon checks the patient's name, the teeth to be extracted, and that there are no dentures or loose teeth and restorations in the mouth. The patient is best treated in the supine position to reduce the risk of fainting during induction. If he is to be seated then the head must be extended so that with the mouth open the mandible is parallel to the ground. With the anaesthetist's agreement a prop, the smallest which will keep the mouth open widely, should be placed as far back in the mouth as possible. A metal or rubber prop is suitable where teeth are present and a rubber McKesson's prop is used between edentulous jaws. The prop must be inspected before it is put in place to ensure it is in good condition and that there is a chain firmly attached to it which can be left hanging out of the mouth (Fig. 13).

When induction is complete the mouth must always be packed with a length of gauze. Several thicknesses of this are placed across the back of the mouth to seal it off from the oropharynx without interfering with the airway. At least 15 cm is left protruding from the mouth for retrieving it in an emergency. Whilst the teeth are being extracted the surgeon must not obstruct the airway, particularly by failing to support the lower jaw. He should beware when extracting from the upper jaw of damaging the lower lip by trapping it between forceps and lower teeth. All broken tooth

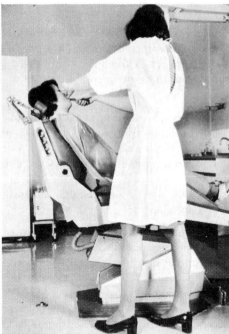

Fig. 28 *Above:* Stance for extracting upper teeth. Note feet apart for steady balance. *Below left:* stance for extracting teeth on lower left, with chair lower than for upper teeth. *Below right:* Position for extracting teeth from lower right quadrant, with operator behind the chair.

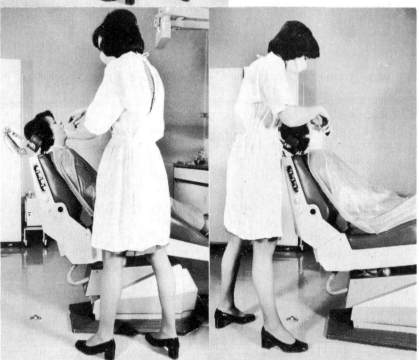

fragments are removed from the mouth immediately, and, together with the extracted teeth, are placed in a special receptacle, care being taken not to carry them back into the mouth by accident.

On finishing the operation the prop and pack are removed by the person who put them in place, and the patient is turned on his side with the lower jaw held forward to allow blood to drain out of the mouth. The mandible is pushed into occlusion to check that the condyles are not dislocated (Chapter XVII). The teeth are counted and all apices checked.

Extractions with the surgeon seated

The chair is adjusted with the patient supine and the surgeon seated on a mobile chair capable of moving in an arc about the patient's head. Only one pattern of lower right-angled premolar forceps is necessary for all extractions in both upper and lower jaws. This is made possible by the use of both hands.

The extractions are performed using the principles described previously in this chapter. The upper and lower teeth on the right side are extracted with the right hand, those on the patient's left with the left hand. Some slight modification of the supporting hand is necessary when working on the upper jaw, but the use of right-angled forceps *does not require any change in the basic movements* used in either jaw (Fig. 29).

Fig. 29 Extraction of teeth with patient supine, showing use of lower right angled premolar forceps to extract upper teeth.

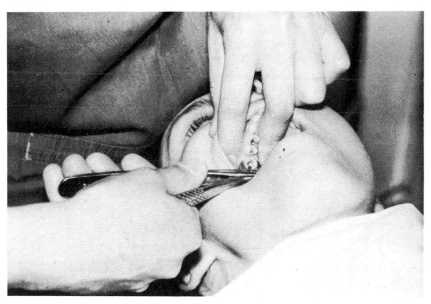

It must be emphasised that there are hazards in operating on a supine patient as displaced teeth, roots or fillings may fall back into the pharynx and the dental surgeon must take adequate steps to prevent this by getting the conscious patient to co-operate by turning his head well to one side during the operation. Further the assistant should have high power suction and a suitable instrument immediately available for grasping any displaced object. Under general anaesthesia the throat must be adequately packed off.

Fracture of the tooth

Fracture of the tooth during extraction occurs frequently, though its incidence may be reduced by a conscientious assessment and a careful progressive technique. Where the fracture is at or above the level of the margin of the alveolar bone and is thought to be due to brittleness or caries and not to excessive resistance, then the extraction may be continued using forceps and elevators as for standing teeth.

In other cases if the fracture is below the level of the alveolar margin or there appears to be undue resistance, the situation should be re-assessed with radiographs. The retained portion may vary in size from a whole root to a tiny apex. It may have broken either before or after there was movement of the tooth. The first decision to be made is whether the root should be left or extracted. There is little doubt that all pieces over 3 mm in length, or those which are non-vital or loose in the socket and might behave as foreign bodies, should be removed. This procedure may be contraindicated if the root lies near some important structure which could be damaged or if there are special medical considerations. Fractured roots of teeth extracted for orthodontic treatment should be removed. Where the orthodontist wishes to move teeth into the extraction site very effort must be made to conserve alveolar bone for this purpose. Whenever it is thought unnecessary or unwise to extract the roots they should be radiographed, the fact noted in the records and *the patient must always be told of their presence.*

Some roots can be seen by direct vision and the operator may decide he can apply elevators or forceps to them successfully through the socket, but often the very limited access makes this difficult and such manipulations can cause considerable trauma to bone and soft tissues. Where the retained fragments cannot be seen by direct vision it is bad surgical practice to attempt them 'blind' and an open or transalveolar approach is required.

The transalveolar approach

This is used to facilitate the extraction of retained roots or teeth which are considered difficult to extract or prove resistant to normal application of forceps or elevators. The surgeon must make a step-by-step plan for this operation, analysing carefully the size of flap, amount of bone removal and the point of application required to deliver the tooth or root satisfactorily.

Fig. 30 Incision for flap for transalveolar approach.

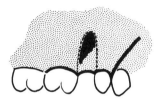

A mucoperiosteal flap is raised to expose the alveolar bone enclosing the retained root. The incision should start at least the width of one tooth behind the root and is carried as far forward again. Where standing teeth are present it is made in the gingival crevice. From its anterior end the incision is then cut obliquely forwards and up or down into the buccal sulcus (Fig. 30). It is designed to avoid dividing the interdental papilla between standing teeth and should lie firmly supported on bone after the root has been removed. Another oblique incision posteriorly may be required to provide adequate access.

Bone is then removed sparingly to expose the root for a few millimetres to provide a new point of application for an elevator mesially, distally or buccally, and to obtain an unobstructed line of withdrawal. An elevator can be used to remove the root. For larger roots a Cryer's elevator can be satisfactorily applied bucally by drilling a hole into the root with a fissure bur at the level of the remaining alveolar bone. This is directed towards the apex at an angle of 45° to allow the elevator a greater range of upward movement (Fig. 31d). Sometimes, where there is hypercementosis or an apical hook, bone may have to be removed down to the apex to free it, care being taken not to expose the roots of neighbouring teeth.

Palatal roots of upper molars do present a problem. When approached buccally it is necessary to remove both the outer alveolar plate and the inter-radicular bone on the buccal aspect of the palatal socket. This gives good access and

Fig. 31 (a) Division of roots of a lower tooth. (b) and (c) Division of upper molar roots. (d) Hole cut to apply Cryer's elevator to buccal aspect of a tooth. Note the angle of the cut to give maximum 'lift' to the root.

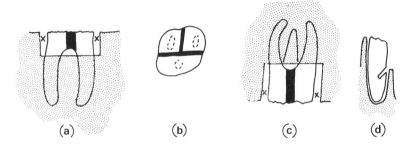

(a)   (b)   (c)   (d)

is a safe approach if the maxillary sinus does not dip down between the roots, but is very extravagant of alveolar bone. A palatal approach is advocated by some but it is more difficult to see into the wound and the bone is quite thick over the apical third of the root. An intra-alveolar approach is probably the best, the interseptal bone between palatal and buccal roots being slowly removed with burs till the root is exposed and an elevator can be used to draw it down.

Where the whole of a difficult tooth or all the roots of an upper or lower molar tooth are retained, the buccal bone should be removed at least to the level of the bifurcation to allow forceps or elevators to be used. A Cryer's elevator may be applied buccally at the bifurcation to lift the roots. In many cases the radiographs will show them to have an unfavourable curvature which requires them to be divided and to be extracted separately (Fig. 31). This may be done with a medium fissure bur. Teeth must not be divided unless they have been exposed sufficiently to leave an adequate point of application on what remains of the roots after division.

A strong word of warning is necessary on two matters. First, the use of elevators on single retained roots which are in close relation to the maxillary sinus, or floor of the nose. *Upward pressure must not be used* even to gain a point of application, as this may cause the root to be displaced into one of these cavities. Bone should be gently removed to expose the root on one surface and downward movements only employed to extract it. In the mandible the inferior dental canal may present a similar hazard. Second, wherever flaps are being raised or bone removed near to the mental foramen the mental nerve must always be found, and preserved. In this respect bone-cutting should be severely limited in the vicinity of this structure.

Removal of roots after the socket has healed

The dental surgeon may be required to extract buried roots as a preparation for dentures, or because they are believed to be a source of pain or sepsis.

Localising roots. Once more diagnosis and assessment is all-important if minimal damage is to be inflicted on the alveolar bone. The first step is to localise the root accurately with two radiographs at right angles to each other; both intraoral apical and occlusal views are required. The antero-posterior position is best established with a localising plate carrying metal markers (Fig. 32). Some surgeons have suggested the use of a suture needle passed through the gum, tied in place to prevent it being swallowed, near the suspected position of the root.

Removal of roots. The principles for removal of old retained roots are the same as for newly fractured teeth. In edentulous jaws the flap may be difficult to reflect and the horizontal incision is best made *just buccal* to the alveolar crest where the mucous membrane is less tightly bound down. Where root apices are deeply placed it is possible to make a curved incision in the alveolus away from the crest of the ridge and remove the fragments through this. Bone is removed sparingly and large roots may be divided to bring

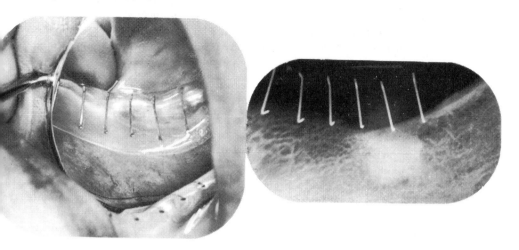

the occlusal portion apically as every attempt must be made to spare the denture-bearing ridge.

Arrest of haemorrhage

After extracting teeth haemorrhage is arrested by asking the patient to bite gently but firmly on the rolled up gauze swab placed over the socket. The buccal and lingual gingival margins of the sockets must not be displaced outward by the swab as this may lead to more bleeding. Should this not stop after ten minutes, digital pressure is applied to the margins of the socket to localise the bleeding point and to confirm that it can be stopped by pressing the gum against the bone. Where this is effective simple interrupted or horizontal mattress sutures are placed across the socket to draw the buccal and lingual alveolar mucoperiosteum together. Though sutures closing an incision should not be tied tightly an exception is post-extraction haemorrhage where the soft tissues must be firmly drawn against the bone. Tight suturing of this kind is contraindicated where a defective clotting mechanism (as in haemophilia) may result in large haemotomas forming in the tissue spaces if the blood is prevented from escaping into the mouth.

Haemorrhage from the vessels in the bony walls of the tooth socket can be controlled by packing with ribbon gauze impregnated with Whitehead's varnish. Care is again taken not to displace the soft tissue margins. The pack is removed a week later.

Agents assisting haemostasis

Vasoconstrictors such as adrenalin 1 : 1000 in distilled water have been applied topically to bleeding wounds. Its use is contraindicated for two reasons. First, once the local effect has worn off it is not unusual to have a reactionary haemorrhage. Second, excess use may result in absorption of appreciable quantities of the adrenalin to give systemic pressure symptoms.

Certain agents assist the physiological clotting mechanism. The most important is thrombin which acts on fibrinogen to form fibrin. Either human or bovine varieties are available and may be applied topically either as a powder or as an aqueous solution on gauze.

Mechanical agents, which include fibrin foam, gelatin foam, oxidised cellulose and oxidised regenerated cellulose, are substances which form a water wettable meshwork and assist clot formation. In general surgery they appear to be readily absorbed from wounds. In oral surgery and especially in tooth sockets they do not seem to behave so well. First, except for oxidised regenerated cellulose, they are difficult to handle and pack into a socket when wet. Second, as the socket is open to the mouth they become contaminated and infected.

Post-extraction instructions

The incidence of post-extraction haemorrhage may be reduced by clear post-extraction instructions (Table 3). The patient must be warned not to use a mouthwash for the first twenty-four hours and thereafter normal oral hygiene may be resumed. Very hot or cold foods, alcohol or exercise are best avoided over the same period. Should bleeding occur he must sit up in bed or on a chair and bite on a rolled-up handkerchief. Where after half an hour these measures fail professional advice is required and he must be given the telephone number and address at which he can contact the dental surgeon. Where extractions were performed under a local anaesthetic the danger of biting or burning the anaesthetised lips or mouth should be stressed, particularly to children.

Further reading

Howe, G. L. (1974), *The Extraction of Teeth*, 2nd edn. John Wright, Bristol.
Lomax, A. M. (1975), 'Extraction techniques for low-seated dentistry', *Brit. Dent. J.*, **138**, 253.

IX Extraction of unerupted teeth

Teeth fail to erupt for many reasons. Evolutionary and hereditary factors which result in a disproportion in size between teeth and jaws are important. Local causes include retention or premature loss of a deciduous predecessor, the presence of supernumerary teeth, abnormal position of or injury to the tooth germ. Tumours and cysts may also prevent teeth from erupting. Certain conditions such as cleft palate, cleidocranial dysostosis, hypopituitarism, cretinism, rickets and facial hemiatrophy predispose to delay or failure of eruption.

The teeth most commonly concerned are the mandibular and maxillary third molars, and the maxillary canine. Others not infrequently seen are the mandibular second premolar and canine, the maxillary central incisors, and supernumerary teeth in both jaws. Many unerupted teeth are impacted – that is, prevented from erupting completely by other teeth or bone. Thus the lower third molar tooth commonly impacts against the second permanent molar.

Reasons for treatment. The majority of unerupted teeth are extracted because they give rise to symptoms of pain or become foci of infection. A number of unerupted teeth, however, are removed because it is obvious they will not come into occlusion and they may disturb the arch or give rise to complications later. In general they are so much easier and safer to remove in young patients that this may justify early prophylactic treatment. Infection is less commonly seen in patients over thirty years old. The removal of asymptomatic unerupted teeth is a difficult decision. The benefits of prophylactic extraction must be balanced against the possible sequelae of the surgery. This is particularly important when considering mandibular premolars and molars where the inferior dental and lingual nerves are at risk.

Diagnosis

The diagnosis of unerupted teeth is based on the history, clinical examination and radiographs.

History

In the absence of infection the patient often has no complaint other than that a tooth is missing. The crown may cause a symptomless swelling under the mucosa. Where pain is thought to be a symptom from a completely buried tooth every effort must be made to eliminate other possible causes particularly pulpitis from another tooth.

Where infection is present more acute symptoms supervene. Inflammation about the crown of an unerupted or partly unerupted tooth is known as pericoronitis and is particularly serious when it arises from a lower third molar owing to the tendency of the infection to spread into the neck (Chapter XII).

Examination

The dentition is accurately charted for missing permanent teeth, retained deciduous teeth, caries and periodontal disease. Caries in a neighbouring tooth can often be the actual cause of the patient's symptoms of pain or infection, or may influence the plan of treatment where extraction of the carious tooth may allow the unerupted one to come into the space. Vitality tests of all doubtful teeth are essential. The unerupted tooth may displace, loosen, or resorb the roots of adjacent teeth against which it impacts. A cyst may form in association with the crown of the buried tooth. (Fig. 33). The mouth is examined for signs of infection such as swelling, discharge, trismus and enlarged tender lymph nodes.

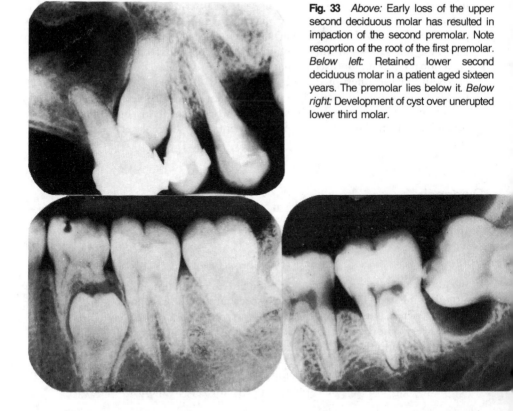

Fig. 33 *Above:* Early loss of the upper second deciduous molar has resulted in impaction of the second premolar. Note resoprtion of the root of the first premolar. *Below left:* Retained lower second deciduous molar in a patient aged sixteen years. The premolar lies below it. *Below right:* Development of cyst over unerupted lower third molar.

Radiography

The object is to show the whole of the unerupted tooth, the size of its crown, and the shape of its roots together with the direction in which they curve. The presence of hypercementosis or widening of the root particularly in the apical third is noted. In multirooted teeth the number of roots and whether they are fused or divergent is important. The position of the tooth in the jaws and its relationship to other teeth including the degree of impaction are an indication of the difficulty of the operation. Secondary conditions such as caries, as increase in the size of the follicle, resorption of adjacent tooth roots or of bone, will all affect the treatment plan (Fig. 33).

Radiographs in two planes at right angles to one another are required to show clearly the position of the tooth and the degree of impaction (Fig. 34). The orthopantomograph is useful as a whole mouth scan where multiple unerupted teeth may be present.

Mandibular teeth.   In the mandible localisation of unerupted teeth must show the whole tooth, its relationship to the inferior dental neurovascular bundle, its buccolingual position, and the relationship to adjacent teeth and the lower border of the mandible. The orthopantomograph is useful to show the position of the inferior dental neurovascular bundle and the depth of the mandible. For lower third molars this may be supplemented by an intraoral periapical film which shows more accurately the morphology of the tooth and its relationship to the second molar. To be of clinical value the radiograph must be correctly taken. The periapical film is placed with the upper border level and parallel with the occlusal plane of the second molar. The central ray is directed so that the buccal and lingual cusps of the second molar are superimposed one upon the other. The contact point between the first and second molars should be clearly shown without overlapping if the central ray has been correctly directed. This ensures that the film shows the true situation at the contact point between the third and second molar teeth, particularly how heavily the former is impacted. The distal bone over the crown of the unerupted tooth should be included. An occlusal film will show the buccolingual positions of buried teeth. It is indicated for those teeth which lie across the arch such as premolars. It is a difficult radiograph to take for third molars.

Deeply placed teeth or those lying in the ascending ramus cannot be seen on intraoral films and if not clearly seen on the orthopantomograph lateral oblique extraoral views may be indicated. These may also be used where there is an extensive secondary condition such as dentigerous cyst or where the mandible is very thin as in elderly edentulous patients.

Where the crown of the third molar tooth has not obviously erupted clear of bone it may be difficult to see on the radiographs exactly how the crown and distal bone are related. If the line of the anterior border of the ascending ramus distal to the third molar is projected to join the margin of the alveolar bone round the second molar, it will give a fair indication of the depth of overlying bone (Fig.35).

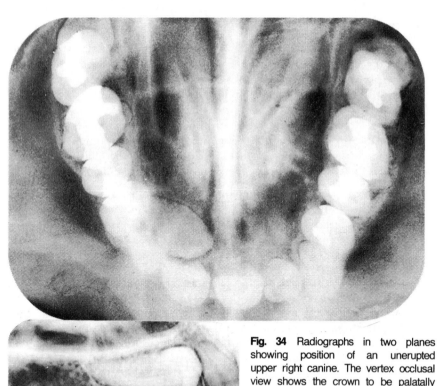

Fig. 34 Radiographs in two planes showing position of an unerupted upper right canine. The vertex occlusal view shows the crown to be palatally placed.

Maxillary teeth. Intraoral periapical and occlusal films are both used in the diagnosis of unerupted maxillary teeth. The maxillary canine may need several periapical films to cover the whole of its length and its relationship to the adjacent teeth. Its position relative to the dental arch is important as it may be placed palatally, buccally, or more rarely across the arch. The only radiograph which will establish the true position of the canine in this respect is the vertex occlusal view taken with the central ray passing through the long axis of the incisor teeth (Fig. 34). This film will also show how close the unerupted canine lies to these teeth and may reveal curvatures of its root not obvious on the periapical view.

Alternatively the parallax method of Clark is used. In this, two periapical radiographs are taken with the films in the same position but with the X-ray tube moved horizontally 3 cm in a known direction between

Fig. 35 Projection of bone over lower third molar. The dotted line is a projection of the anterior border of the ascending ramus extended to join the margin of the alveolar bone distal to the second molar, indicating that the distal cusp of the third molar is just covered by bone.

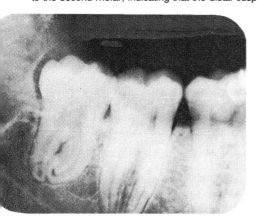 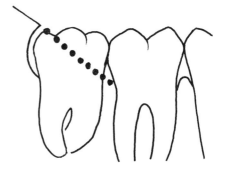

exposures (that is from 1.5 cm behind the normal centring point to 1.5 cm in front of it). Where two teeth lie in different planes the one which appears to move in the same direction as the X-ray tube lies furthest from it, that is palatally. In analysing these radiographs the relationship of the crown and the root of the buried tooth to the roots of the standing teeth must be considered separately.

The true position of the unerupted tooth in the vertical dimension is not accurately shown on a periapical film because of the angle at which the ray is directed onto the maxilla. The orthopantomograph may provide a more satisfactory answer and will show unerupted teeth high in the maxilla related to the maxillary sinus. In teeth lying buccal to the arch a tangential view of the maxilla may be of assistance. Other unerupted maxillary teeth, supernumerary teeth and mesiodens are examined radiographically in much the same way.

Summary of findings

From his investigations the dental surgeon should know the following facts about the patient and the unerupted tooth. The patient's age, general development and the state of the dentition; the size and form of the crown of the unerupted tooth; whether it is resorbed or, in partly erupted teeth, carious; the form of the roots, fused or divergent, straight, or curved mesially or distally. The position of the tooth in the bone, whether it is lying vertically, horizontally or inverted, how deeply it is buried in bone and its buccolingual or palatal relation to the arch. The relationship of the tooth to other teeth and to vital structures such as nerves, the nose and the maxillary sinus. The size of the follicle which may have atrophied, making extraction more difficult, undergone cystic change or have become infected. The texture of the bone, signs of osteosclerosis or in edentulous patients the degree of resorption of the mandible. The state of the adjoining teeth, whether caries, periodontal disease, apical areas or root resorption are present. With these facts established treatment may now be considered.

Treatment

Treatment may be either conservative, to bring the tooth into useful occlusion in the arch, or by extraction.

Conservative treatment

Conservative treatment should be considered for patients where the tooth might be brought into occlusion. The advice of a specialist orthodontist is necessary as orthodontic treatment may be required prior to surgery to create space in the arch for the unerupted tooth. A conservative approach is particularly important where a neighbouring standing tooth is carious or heavily filled. In some cases eruption may not take place without exposure of the tooth and the use of traction.

Exposure of teeth. To expose teeth a mucoperiosteal flap is made, bone is removed with burs to free the crown down to its greatest circumference. For incisors and canines the cingulum must be exposed. Every precaution should be taken to avoid dislodging the tooth accidentally. Where the orthodontist wants a bracket, or other device to apply traction, this is placed at operation. For palatally placed teeth the soft tissues are then excised round the crown and the dead space packed with Coepack or Whitehead's varnish on gauze. These are removed after ten days when the patient should be referred back to the orthodontist. Care must be taken with exposure of buccally placed teeth for there is evidence that excision of the soft tissues back to non-keratinised mucosa results in an unsatisfactory epithelial cuff around the erupted tooth. Many orthodontists prefer to apply a bracket to such teeth with a wire brought out through the wound for traction. The mucoperiosteal flap is then sutured back into position.

Surgical repositioning and transplantion

In both these techniques the tooth, after exposure, is moved bodily to bring it into the dental arch. In surgical repositioning the tooth is rotated through an angle which must be less than 90 to prevent damage to the apical vessels. In transplantation the tooth is carefully extracted and placed in a surgically prepared socket. It is immobilised with a splint for about four weeks when it is usually firm. The teeth most frequently transplanted are unerupted maxillary canines replanted into their correct position and third molars used to replace carious first molars. Good results are obtained with young patients, but resorption of roots is a complication after two to five years which occasionally leads to loss of the tooth.

Extraction of unerupted teeth

Where the unerupted tooth cannot be treated conservatively extraction is best performed early in life before it is complicated by sclerosis of bone, atrophy of the follicle which reduces the free space round the crown, or by the presence of infection. The roots when fully formed frequently develop hooked or bulbous apices and in adults the impaction of the crown against adjoining teeth is often severe.

Ideally the tooth is removed when the roots are two-thirds complete; before this the crown may be difficult to elevate as it tends to turn in its socket like the ball in a ball-and-socket joint. Removal of a symptomless tooth is best postponed if it is acting as a buttress for the root of an adjacent tooth which may be simultaneously bereft of support and denuded of bone.

It is also contraindicated where vital structures such as the inferior dental nerve may be damaged in the course of operation. In acute pericoronitis surgery must be delayed until the acute phase has settled.

Planning the operation. This is best done by considering *first* the position of the tooth in the jaw, *second* its natural line of withdrawal, *third* the obstacles to its extraction and how these may best be overcome, *fourth* the points of application for elevators, and *finally* access by removing bone and raising the flap sufficient to allow the necessary procedures to be performed.

Thus the plan is made in the *reverse order* to that in which the operation will be performed as obviously the size and form of the flap depends on bone removal and this in turn is related to the position of the tooth and any manoeuvres required to disimpact it.

Natural line of withdrawal. This may be shown on radiographs by projecting the line along which the tooth would move if it followed the course dictated by the curvature of its roots. Teeth are most easily extracted by moving them out of their sockets or out of bone along this pathway. Where the tooth would come through the alveolus into the mouth unimpeded, except by alveolar bone, it is said to be favourably placed, but where it would go deeper into bone or impact against another tooth it is classified as unfavourable.

Extraction by moving the teeth along their line of withdrawal is done with elevators, using a gentle touch and always watching the effect of the forces applied to the tooth or roots. Heavy levering either to disimpact the tooth or lift it from its socket may have serious consequences such as fracture of the bone, or displacement of the tooth into the soft tissues or the maxillary sinus. Where the roots of mandibular teeth are near the inferior dental canal this nerve may be damaged. Resistance to elevation should be foreseen and plans made to overcome it.

Obstacles to elevation of a tooth. They may occur along its natural line of withdrawal and may be 'intrinsic', that is due to the shape of the tooth, such as hooked or bulbous apices, roots curving in opposite directions, or a constriction at the neck of the tooth all of which may anchor the tooth in bone. As many of these difficulties are found in the apical third of the root considerable bone removal may be necessary to free the tooth.

The obstacles may also be 'extrinsic', that is due to bone, adjacent teeth or vital structures such as the inferior dental nerve or the maxillary antrum. The depth of the tooth in bone is a major factor in assessing difficulty, presenting problems of access, increasing the time of operation, and requiring foresight and experience to avoid excessive bone destruction.

Where the unerupted tooth is impacted against other teeth which are not for extraction its disimpaction is usually a simple problem in geometry. The tooth may be extracted whole by removing sufficient bone to allow it to be rotated, and this is often possible (Fig. 36a). Where the impaction is severe (Fig. 36e) or the root curvature adverse (Fig. 36b) it must be divided and extracted in pieces. This is a less traumatic and safer method than forceful levering to disimpact the tooth and preserves bone which may later form part of the edentulous denture-bearing ridge. Division may be horizontal (crown from roots, Fig. 36e) or vertical (down the long axis of the tooth, Fig. 36d). Both are preferably done with a large bur, to leave an appreciable space between the divided parts. A hole is made through the centre of the root below the amelocemental junction with a No. 7 fissure

Fig. 36 The distal bone to be removed is shown by cross-hatching. (a) Mesioangular impaction with favourable roots. The tooth will rotate about the apex of the distal root to disimpact the crown. (b) Mesioangular impaction with unfavourable roots requiring division. (c) Distoangular impaction with oblique division to leave point of application (X). (d) Vertical impaction with unfavourable roots requiring vertical division. (e) Horizontal impaction. Note angulation of cut to allow disimpaction of the crown distally up the inclined plane. (f) Forward elevation of the root showing the point of application against the distal bone.

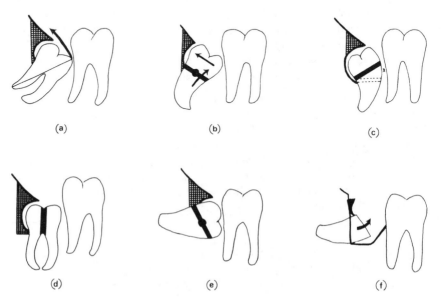

(a) (b) (c)

(d) (e) (f)

bur. To divide the crown from the roots the cut is extended mesially and distally through the whole thickness of the tooth. The angle of cut is important and should be made to favour the line of withdrawal of the crown (Fig. 36 and 37). Wherever the tooth is related to any important structure a thick layer of dentine is left intact and the last portion cracked through by rotating an elevator in the cut. Division with an osteotome is less satisfactory as it produces a hair-line crack, often at the wrong angle, which makes disimpaction of the crown very difficult. When it is used, the tooth must be firmly supported in bone and not loose; the osteotome is applied to the cementum and given a sharp blow with the mallet.

Division vertically is reserved for molar teeth, particularly those with divergent roots, and is very effective in certain impactions (Fig. 36d). It is obviously ineffective where the roots are fused or the cut misses their bifurcation. Removal of part of the crown has been advocated in the literature but has little advantage over horizontal division, though it may sometimes leave a convenient point of application for an elevator (Fig. 36c).

Point of application for elevators.   Dental elevators when properly used are very sensitive instruments through which even the slightest resistance to movement of a tooth or root can be felt. For this reason they are the most satisfactory instrument for extracting buried teeth. It must be decided at the planning stage at which points it will be necessary to apply an elevator to lift the tooth, or after it has been divided the crown and then the roots, out of the socket. Bone may have to be removed with the sole object of obtaining satisfactory access or a fulcrum for the elevator. Tooth division must be planned so that after removal of the crown enough root is exposed to enable elevators to be applied easily. No tooth should be divided until an adequate point of application on the fraction that is to be left in bone has been prepared and tested otherwise the operator's difficulties may be greatly increased by his injudicious action.

Fig. 37 Impacted second premolar: (a) bone removal, and division of tooth; (b) correct buccolingual angulation of the dividing cut; (c) incorrect angulation as crown cannot disimpact from the first molar.

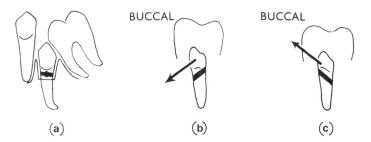

(a)   (b)   (c)

Access. Only after all the above factors have been considered can the full extent of bone removal be calculated. Inadequate access is the commonest cause of difficulty in the extraction of unerupted teeth. The flap must be sufficiently large to allow direct vision into the whole field. Bone removal should permit the greatest circumference of the crown to pass freely out of the bone along the planned line of withdrawal and provide access for dividing the tooth if necessary. Where the greatest diameter of the roots is not at the neck of the tooth, the bulbous section must be made free of bone. The cutting of bone should not be punctuated by hopeful attempts to extract the tooth, but is completed as one stage of the operation before elevation is tried. Indeed the preparation of satisfactory access for elevators and of a fulcrum on firm bone offering them adequate support is an important part of planned bone removal.

The size and shape of the flap in its turn depends on the extent of the operation as it must provide access without subjecting the soft tissues to tension or trauma. The flap must extend beyond the area of bone removal so that the line of closure rests on bone.

Teeth in edentulous jaws. These often present in older patients when the bone is sclerotic and the periodontal space very narrow. The principles of removal are similar to those described, but it may be necessary to cut a point of application for an elevator and very gentle forces should be applied as the bone is brittle. Special care is taken to preserve the alveolar ridge by making an accurate assessment and removing minimal bone. Where gross resorption of the mandible has taken place, and there is danger of fracturing the jaw, the patient should be warned and splints constructed before the operation.

Closure. Debridement is completed in the normal way and the flap reapposed. Sutures are tied loosely and no attempt should be made to close any soft tissue deficiency present before operation by reason of a partly erupted tooth.

Extraction of the unerupted lower third molar

Assessment

Position of the tooth and its line of withdrawal. The position of the unerupted lower third molar may be vertical (Fig. 36d), horizontal (Fig. 36e), mesioangular (Fig. 36a) or distoangular (Fig. 36c). The crown usually lies nearer the lingual than the buccal plate. Occasionally it is inverted or lies across the mandible, with the crown facing either bucally or lingually. Very rarely it is found in the ascending ramus or at the lower border of the mandible. Where the tooth lies below the inferior dental canal an extraoral lower border approach is indicated.

The natural line of the tooth can only be determined by a study of radiographs showing the form of the roots which may be fused, divergent, straight or curved to favour or prevent extraction of the tooth.

The difficulty of the extraction is increased if access is difficult. This may occur if the mouth is small, where the space between the anterior border of the mandible and the distal aspect of the second molar is narrow or when the tooth is deeply buried in bone.

Obstacles to extraction

Bone. All or part of the crown may be covered by bone (Fig. 35). How deeply the tooth is buried is calculated by measuring the vertical distance from the cervical margin of the second molar to the mesial cervical margin of the tooth except in distoangular impactions where the distal cervical margin is used. Where this distance is over 4 mm the tooth should be regarded as deeply buried. Vertically placed buried teeth may only need bone to be removed from over the whole of the occlusal and buccal surfaces of the crown for them to be elevated up and out with a Cryer's elevator applied to the buccal aspect of the root.

They must, however, be distinguished from the tooth that is distally impacted against the bone of the ascending ramus. These are the most difficult of all impacted third molars to extract. They should always be approached with great caution, especially where they are deeply placed, lie far back in the ascending ramus, or the roots have a distal curvature (Fig. 36c).

After removal of buccal and occlusal bone to clear the crown the tooth should be divided, the crown removed, and using a point of application on the buccal aspect of the roots they are elevated into the space created.

Where the roots are curved distally this may still prove difficult until further bone has been cut to free them distally, or the roots are sectioned again. If the roots are separate vertical division is often useful.

The inferior dental neurovascular bundle. This may be damaged by direct trauma from burs or elevators, or indirectly when the tooth is elevated or rotated as the root can crush or tear the neurovascular bundle.

The relationship of roots, particularly of the lower third molar, to the inferior dental canal may be deduced from radiographs. It may clearly lie below the roots or appear to cross them. In the latter relationship it is probably grooving the roots if the radiolucent band of the canal is seen to cross them above their apices. Where the root is deeply notched the white lines, representing the cortical plates lining the canal, converge, are diverted or interrupted (Fig. 38). This is a warning that heavy or repeated elevation may compress the nerve against bone to cause hypoaesthesia or paraesthesia. Such damage can be avoided by planning the operation so that sufficient bone is removed and, where indicated, the tooth divided to allow the roots to be lifted out with a single gentle movement.

Perforation of a root by the canal contents is suggested where the radiolucent band crosses the root and shows the loss of both white lines with maximum constriction of the radiolucent band at the middle of the root (Fig. 38d). The tooth must then be divided, and removed from around the nerve or,

Fig. 38 Relationship of the third molar roots to the inferior dental canal as seen on radiographs: (a) root lightly notched; (b) apical notch; (c) deeply notched; (d) the canal perforates the root.

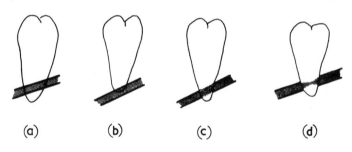

(a)   (b)   (c)   (d)

where this is not possible, the nerve is cut with a sharp scalpel and the ends replaced in the canal, following which, sensation often returns after a few months.

Impaction against a tooth. The third molar may impact against the second molar either in the mesioanglar (Fig. 36a) or in the horizontal position (Fig. 36e). The impaction may be overcome in one of three ways.

Extraction of the second molar can be justified by gross caries or periodontal disease. It is often advised where the third molar is heavily impacted against the distal root of the second molar without any apparent intervening alveolar bone. This should not be necessary if the surgeon avoids damaging the second molar roots and the soft tissue round the neck of that tooth. Usually the second molar is sound and the operation must be planned to protect it from damage during the extraction of the buried tooth.

Rotation of the impacted tooth, particularly if it is in a favourable mesioangular position, may allow it to be turned bodily away from the second molar. This can be planned on radiographs. The apex of the distal root of the third molar is taken as the centre of a circle through which the tooth might be rotated. A radius is drawn to the mesiobuccal cusp and if the arc of this circle passes clear of the second molar, then the third molar should disimpact without difficulty, providing sufficient bone can be removed distally to allow it to turn (Fig. 36a). This technique is often satisfactory for mesioangular impactions, but would require extensive bone removal for horizontal impactions. When assessing the tooth for rotation the relationship of the apex of the distal root to the inferior dental canal should be examined as rotation may force this apex downwards and if the canal is immediately below, the neurovascular bundle may be crushed with resulting anaesthesia or paraesthesia.

Division of the impacted tooth is indicated where the impaction is heavy, the curvature of the roots is unfavourable or where a large amount of bone would otherwise have to be removed. In horizontal impactions bone is removed from the buccal and upper surface of the crown and coronal third of the root. The tooth is then divided through the neck, using an oblique cut (Fig. 37e) so that the crown may be easily disimpacted by sliding it up and back along the distally inclined plane on the root. The roots are then brought forward using a Cryer's elevator on their superior surface. Where the roots have a mesial unfavourable curvature or are divergent, difficulty may be experienced and further division of the roots may be necessary.

Operative technique

The flap. The incision for partly erupted third molars is commenced in the distal part of the gingival crevice and carried buccally round the crown of the tooth to just behind the crown of the second molar (where the tooth is buried the incision starts on the alveolar crest, distal to the second molar). It is then carried down and slightly anteriorly to the reflection where it is turned to run forward parallel to, but just above the reflection, stopping just short of the distal root of the first molar, to avoid a small artery at this point. Using a Mitchell's trimmer the edge of the flap is freed starting in the buccal sulcus and working distally. It may then be reflected with the Howarth's periosteal elevator to expose the external oblique line of the mandible. The incision is then continued along this line and up the ascending ramus using either scissors or a scalpel on the anterior edge of the ramus where the flap will fall away from the bone easily and small vessels are avoided (Fig. 39).

The buccal and lingual flaps are then reflected to expose the lingual, occlusal and buccal aspects of the retromolar triangle. This may be difficult where the flap is closely attached to the third molar follicle. The lingual flap is reflected using a Howarth's periosteal elevator in a distolingual direction. Care must be taken to ensure that the periosteum is reflected from the bone and not split as it curves over the lingual bony ridge. Damage to the lingual nerve which lies between the lingual periosteum and mucosa is thus avoided.

Bone removal. This can be done in several ways. Bone may be removed to expose the buried tooth by grinding it away using rosehead or fissure burs. A guttering technique has been suggested but has certain disadvantages in that access and visibility are not good and distolingual bone is retained. Further, the buccal cortical plate is left with a very poor blood supply as it is stripped of periosteum on the side the flap has been raised and of vascular cancellous bone by the bur on the other side. Finally the thin wall of bone is easily crushed by elevators when extracting the tooth.

The collar technique designed for use with burs is a modification of Sir William Kelsey Fry's split bone technique. It has the advantage that the calculated amount of bone can be removed as a block, including the distolingual angle of bone which so often prevents satisfactory distal rotation of the mesioangular impacted tooth. It can be used to expose horizontally impacted teeth but is not suitable for relieving distoangular impactions.

Fig. 39 Incision for extraction of unerupted third molar. The distal extension (dotted line) follows the external oblique ridge of the mandible.

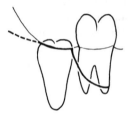

Bone removal is performed with a No. 5 fissure bur. The first cut starts distal to the second molar and is taken downwards. Its length is such that it ends at the proposed point of application for an elevator, on the mesial cervical margin of the lower third molar. The bur is then moved distally at this level making sure that the full depth of buccal plate is cut through. When the distal aspect of the buried tooth is reached the cut continues backwards for 2 mm and is then curved distally and lingually until it just penetrates the lingual plate (Fig. 40). In the last phase the bur lies across the mandible behind the buried tooth. The distal cut is then deepened by moving the bur downwards and forwards until it reaches the distal aspect of the tooth. This is most important. The tooth is now surrounded by a collar of bone which is only attached to the mandible by its lingual plate. A Coupland's elevator is placed towards the lingual side of the distal cut and rotated gently. This will cause the lingual plate to fracture at the point where it is thinned by the crown of the tooth and the whole collar of bone is lifted out of the wound leaving the crown of the tooth exposed (Fig. 40). Horizontally impacted teeth may then be divided whereas mesioangular teeth are disimpacted using a No. 1 Coupland's elevator or a straight Warwick James elevator placed mesially, at the neck of the tooth, and rotated to move it distally and lingually, it is then lifted out of its socket with a Cryer's elevator used mesially or buccally in the bifurcation of the roots.

Fig. 40 Bone removal for collar technique. (a) Buccal cut made with bur and extended distally through the lingual plate, (b) Vertical view of cut, with arrow to show point at which the thin lingual plate fractures. (c) Collar of bone removed exposing crown with sufficient space to disimpact the tooth distally.

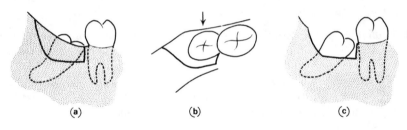

(a) (b) (c)

Debridement. The wound must be cleansed of debris and the follicle of the tooth removed by grasping it firmly in tissue forceps and drawing it gently off the bone. Where it is attached to the flap, this may be gently dissected off with a Mitchell's trimmer.

Closure. One suture in the distal part of the incision, over the external oblique ridge, is usually sufficient to hold the flap in position. No attempt should be made to pull the flap across a deficiency created by a partially erupted tooth.

Extraction of the upper third molar tooth

Assessment. Access is made difficult by the position of the upper third molar behind the second molar, the presence of the malar buttress, and the way in which the coronoid process comes forward when the mouth is open. Fortunately, the majority are buccally placed and covered by only a thin layer of bone.

Their roots vary widely in form but they are often small and fine and fracture easily. The roots, and sometimes the whole tooth, are commonly in close relation to the maxillary sinus into which they can be displaced. Deeply placed distoangular teeth can easily be pushed into the soft tissue behind the maxillary tuberosity. Upper third molars seldom give trouble whilst buried and in view of this there is a strong argument for leaving those that are symptomless to erupt or until the second molar is to be extracted. Erupted upper third molars which are functionless should be extracted at the same time as the lower third molar.

The flap. The incision is made from the distal aspect of the maxillary tuberosity forward to the middle of the distal aspect of the second molar crown. This part of the incision should be kept over towards the palate to expose the third molar without raising a second palatal flap which is often difficult to retract and may cause retching in some patients. The incision is then taken round the neck of the second molar and carried obliquely· forward into the buccal sulcus. The flap is reflected and held back with the periosteal elevator (Fig. 41).

Bone removal. The bone over this tooth is usually quite thin and can be removed with burs or with a sharp chisel used with gentle pressure by hand to avoid accidentally pushing the tooth into the maxillary sinus. When the occlusal, buccal and distal aspect of the crown have been exposed an elevator (Cryer's or Warwick James) may be applied to the buccal surface of this tooth to bring it *downwards*. Mesioangular impactions may be disimpacted from behind the upper second molar with an elevator. In either case a Howarth's raspatory must be placed distally to prevent the tooth being luxated backward into the soft tissues (Fig. 41).

Fig. 41 (a) Design of buccal flap for upper third molar. Note that the distal extension of the incision over the tuberosity is carried well over towards the palatal side. (b) Extraction of upper third molar with a Howarth's raspatory placed behind the tooth to prevent it displacing backwards into the soft tissue spaces.

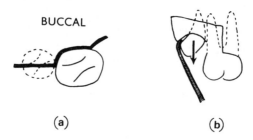

BUCCAL

(a)   (b)

Extraction of the unerupted maxillary canine

Assessment. The unerupted maxillary canine may lie palatally, bucally or across the dental arch between the roots of the standing teeth. In this last case the root apex or the crown may be palpated in the buccal sulcus. Some are deeply placed high up in the maxilla or in the floor of the nose. The tooth may be in vertical, mesioangular, distoangular, or horizontal impaction; rarely it is inverted. Many unerupted canines have curved roots often sharply hooked in the apical third.

Radiographs in two planes must be carefully examined to localise the tooth, to determine its relationship to the dental arch and to detect the site and direction of any curvature of the roots (Fig. 34). The relationship of the canine to the standing teeth is most important, particularly for palatally placed canines which may in fact have caused so much resorption of alveolar bone that they are supporting the teeth against which they are impacted. Wherever the impaction is close, or the standing teeth have been moved or show signs of resorption by the canine, vitality tests should be carried out, and splints prepared beforehand to support the standing teeth during and after operation.

In those canines lying in the arch between the roots of the standing teeth tangential views of the maxilla are important in determining the position of the incisal tip, whether it is lying palatal or buccal to the arch. Where it has passed buccally between the roots of the teeth it is necessary to expose the crown buccally even though the tooth may have to be approached palatally as well.

It is a common fault for inexperienced surgeons to omit to make a stage-by-stage operation plan for unerupted canines, possibly because the approach to these teeth is less standardised than for the lower third molar. It is essential before starting to be quite clear about the proposed line of withdrawal, the bone to be removed and the points of application to be prepared.

Buccally placed canines

These are extracted through a buccal incision, which is made in a long curve about 3 cm in length and at least half a centimetre above the gingival margin of the standing teeth. The thin layer of bone over the tooth is removed and it is gently eased outwards with a Cryer's elevator and, when it is disimpacted, extracted with forceps.

Palatally placed canines

The flap. As the approach is through a palatal flap the field of operation is best seen if the surgeon works from the opposite side, that is the patient's left, for a tooth on the right. The incision is made in the gingival crevice round the necks of the standing teeth. For a tooth on the right side it extends from the upper left canine to the upper right first molar. The flap is reflected carefully to lift the mucoperiosteum containing the palatine artery without damaging that vessel. The structures passing through the incisive foramen are divided as they restrict access (Fig. 42a).

Where two canines are to be extracted the flap is best made from first molar to first molar. The flap can be held back with a retractor, a hook or by passing a suture though it tied to the teeth on the opposite side.

Bone removal. This should be done very accurately with a medium-sized rosehead bur (5–9) keeping *to the palatal side* of the buried tooth. Bone is removed till the crown is found; it is then cleared of bone particularly over the incisive tip and the coronal third of the root. Every effort must be made to *leave the supporting bone over the roots of the standing teeth* and to avoid accidentally cutting into their roots. Special care is needed where the canine lies across the arch.

Fig. 42 (*a*) Design of a palatal flap for extraction of a buried canine. Note the position of the incisive foramen and the palatine vessels. (*b*) Palatal flap reflected and upper left canine being extracted using a Coupland's elevator.

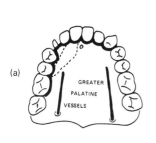

(a)

GREATER
PALATINE
VESSELS

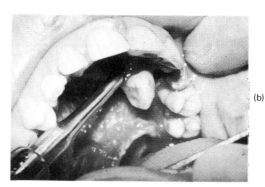

(b)

Extraction. Many vertical canines with straight roots will elevate downwards once the crown is cleared. Others, particularly those in a horizontal position impacted against other teeth, should be divided and the crown extracted first. Elevators are best applied to the palatal side of the tooth or up its long axis. Occasionally, elevation from the buccal side is unavoidable. In these circumstances the fingers of the watching hand are placed over the standing teeth to detect even the slightest movement in them, and, where a splint has been constructed this may be put over the teeth to support them and removed after the extraction.

Great difficulty may be found when the apical third of the root is curved or hooked, particularly if this curvature is unfavourable and turns the tooth into the dental arch, making it necessary to remove bone from over its whole length to free the apex. Many canines are closely related to the maxillary sinus into which they can be displaced by forceful or misdirected application of elevators. Should a root apex which is known to be near the antrum fracture it is wise to consider leaving it.

Those teeth which lie across the dental arch with the crown in the palate and the root apex in the buccal sulcus may require a flap made both palatally and buccally. Where the apex of the root is hooked, division may be necessary to extract the apex bucally, and to allow the crown to be removed palatally which can often be done by firm pressure exerted through the buccal approach.

Closure. The palatal flap when replaced will require only one or two sutures to hold it. The knots should be tied buccally.

Osteoplastic flaps. Canines in edentulous jaws are often lying along the arch so that their removal may destroy the bony ridge and damage the denture bearing area. The ridge can be preserved by the use of an osteoplastic flap. Two buccal, vertical incisions are made just beyond the estimated position of the root apex and the incisal tip of the tooth. These are joined by an incision along the crest of the ridge. The margin, 3 mm only, of the buccal flap is reflected to admit a chisel or fissure bur which is used to make cuts through the bone parallel to the vertical and horizontal incisions. The latter must be on the crest of the ridge and cut up to the

Fig. 43 Osteoplastic flap. *Left:* Continuous dark line indicates the incision through mucoperiosteum along the alveolar crest and extended obliquely upwards in the buccal mucoperiosteum anteriorly and posteriorly. Dashed line indicates limited extent of reflection of the flap to allow bone incision to be made. *Right:* Mucoperiosteum and bone flap reflected to expose canine tooth.

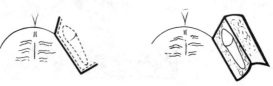

Fig. 44 Supernumerary teeth. *Above:* Radiograph showing multiple supernumeraries in the incisor region. *Below:* Same case after operation.

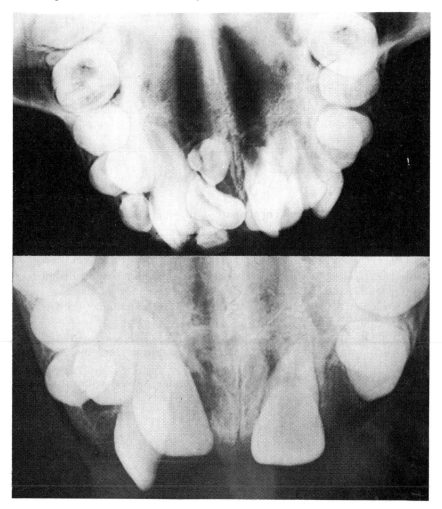

tooth. A Howarth's periosteal elevator is placed in this cut and rotated outwards so that the buccal bone fractures and, still attached to mucoperiosteum, is raised buccally (Fig. 43). The canine can then be seen and removed with an elevator. The osteoplastic flap is carefully replaced and the mucosa sutured. The bony ridge is thus preserved and the patient can often continue to wear the denture within alteration.

Extraction of maxillary supernumerary teeth

Supernumerary teeth in the incisor region of the maxilla are of common occurrence. They are diagnosed and operated in much the same way as unerupted maxillary canines. Where the supernumerary is associated with an unerupted incisor it is best extracted as soon as possible to avoid causing delayed or arrested eruption. It is essential to expose clearly and identify the permanent teeth and the supernumerary *without doubt* before any form of elevation is started.

Other unerupted teeth

Other unerupted teeth in the maxilla and mandible will present their own problems to the surgeon which he must solve by applying the principles described above to each new situation.

Further reading

Hitchen, A. D. (1955), 'The impacted maxillary canine', *Brit. Dent. J.*, **100**, 1.

Hitchin, A. D. (1966), 'The unerupted mandibular premolar', *Brit. Dent. J.*, **120**, 117.

Howe, G. L. (1985), *Minor Oral Surgery*, 3rd edn. John Wright, Bristol.

Howe, G. L. and Poyton, H. G. (1960), 'Prevention of damage to the inferior dental nerve during the extraction of mandibular third molar', *Brit. Dent. J.*, **109**, 335.

Rood, J. P. and Nooraldeen Shehab, B.A.A. (1990), 'The radiological prediction of inferior alveolar nerve injury during third molar surgery, *Brit. J.O.M. Surg.*, **28**, 20.

Ward, T. G. (1965), 'The split bone technique for the removal of lower third molars', *Brit. Dent. J.*, **101**, 297.

x Complications of tooth extraction

Difficulty of access

Trismus. Limitation of opening may be due to intrinsic causes (abnormalities in the temporomandibular joint) or extrinsic causes (facial scars and inflammatory swellings). In chronic cases it may be possible to improve the opening with exercisers, but forcing the jaws open when trismus is due to infection will break down the pyogenic membrane and cause spread. The acute phase is treated with antibiotics and drainage and the extractions delayed till the opening is sufficiently improved.

Reduced aperture of the mouth. This may be due to congenital malformation (microstomia) or to scarring, making it difficult or even impossible to apply forceps or elevators to the teeth. In extreme cases a surgical approach through the angle of the mouth may be necessary.

Crowded or misplaced teeth. These frequently make it difficult to apply forceps or elevators without the risk of loosening adjacent teeth. This may be made easier by dividing or grinding down, with discs or burs, the tooth to be extracted.

Abnormal resistance

Where there is no obvious clinical cause for abnormal resistance such as the position of the tooth or the thickness of the alveolar bone, the operator should make steady and repeated efforts to loosen the tooth, avoiding too much force in one direction. After a reasonable attempt, if there is no movement, a radiograph is taken before proceeding further. This may show abnormalities of the roots in number or in form such as twisted, divergent, bulbous or hypercementosed roots. In age or chronic periodontal disease there may be sclerosis of the alveolar bone. Isolated teeth in occlusion are renownedly difficult to remove owing to narrowing of the periodontal membrane, Unerupted teeth impacting against the roots of the tooth to be extracted (lower third molar against second molar roots) can be a source of difficulty only discovered on a radiograph.

In all cases of abnormal resistance it is advisable to plan removal of the tooth through a transalveolar approach to reduce trauma and avoid fracturing the tooth.

Damage to other teeth

Extraction of the wrong tooth. This is a common source of litigation and is indefensible because it is avoidable if the proper precautions are taken. Extractions should never be started without checking *immediately* before operation, the patient's name, address and age, the teeth to be removed and any radiographs available. This applies equally to patients operated upon under local or general anaesthesia. The patient, or in the case of children the parent, is asked to confirm he understands which teeth are to be extracted, and any doubts in his mind must be settled before the anaesthetic is given.

The notes should be placed so that the operator can see them throughout the operation and can make a final check just before the forceps are applied to the tooth. Should an error occur, the surgeon must proceed to extract the right tooth to complete the operation. He has then to decide whether to re-implant the wrongly extracted tooth immediately or to accept the situation.

Dislocation of adjacent teeth or of restorations in adjacent teeth. Careless application or movements of forceps and elevators may cause this mishap. Forceps can accidentally engage part of the next tooth and so loosen it, or when drawing a lower tooth from its socket without sufficient control they may bang against the upper teeth. Elevators, misused either as class I levers or by employing a neighbouring tooth, and not bone, as the fulcrum, can do similar damage. The watching fingers of the supporting hand can assist in preventing this by feeling that the forceps are in good position and detecting even slight movement in adjacent teeth. Where misplaced or mildly impacted teeth occur in the arch a disc or bur should be used on the tooth to allow of its extraction without transmitting pressure or force to its neighbours.

The permanent premolars may be luxated when extracting the deciduous molars due to the root formation of the deciduous teeth which may closely approximate the crown of the permanent tooth, or infection which may cause fibrosis or even ankylosis between them. More often it is due to the misapplication of instruments in the extraction of deciduous molars or injudicious attempts to remove their retained roots.

Fracture of teeth

Where normal extracting methods are used the teeth may fracture owing to advanced caries or large restorations which weaken the crown. In devitalised teeth, in periodontal disease and in the aged, the roots may become brittle, and it is unfortunate that the last two conditions are also characterised by sclerosis and loss of elasticity of the alveolar bone thereby causing undue resistance to add to the dentist's difficulties.

Another common cause is ill-fitting forceps which impinge on the crown or do not fit the root accurately. Forceps may be misapplied particularly on rotated, inclined or misplaced teeth. The use of excess force or short, jerky movements prevent the surgeon feeling which way the tooth wants to come and frequently result in fracture.

The management of retained roots has been discussed in Chapter VIII. However, if certain principles are neglected their attempted removal may lead to more serious complications. It is essential that a radiograph should be taken and, except where the crown has fractured at or above the level of the alveolar margin, it is bad practice to use forceps up the socket as the limited access makes it difficult to open the beaks sufficiently to grasp the root. Only too often they are applied knowing that one or both blades are outside the alveolus which must be crushed to deliver the root. The transalveolar approach must always be used wherever the root is not clearly visible or supporting tissues will be damaged. It is safe, leaves the tissue in good condition, and, if regularly practised without delay, is economic in time.

Loss of tooth or roots

As the teeth and roots are extracted they should be carefully placed in a special container, care being taken not to carry them back into the mouth by accident. At the end of the operation, particularly under general anaesthesia, they should be counted and the number checked against the chart.

Where during extractions a tooth or root is lost, the surgeon should *immediately* stop operating and conduct a systematic search.

The mouth. All the recesses of the mouth, under the tongue and recent sockets are examined. In patients under general anaesthesia, the posterior aspect of the tongue and oropharynx are searched too. After this has been done the superficial layers of the throat pack may be drawn forward lest it be lying there. The pack should not be removed completely till the end of the operation.

Spittoon and suction apparatus. The spittoon should always have a trap, and the suction apparatus a bottle in the circuit to stop fragments of tooth disappearing down the drain. The sucker head, rubber tubing and other connections should be washed through as they often trap root apices.

Alimentary tract or lungs. Roots or teeth may be swallowed or inhaled. Whenever it is suspected that this may have happened radiographs of the chest or abdomen should be taken. Swallowed fragments seldom give cause for anxiety, though their passage through the gut should be monitored, but if inhaled into the lungs the patient must be referred, without delay, to a thoracic surgeon for removal by bronchoscopy.

Under the mucoperiosteum. Roots and occasionally teeth can be displaced under the periosteum particularly in the mandible where there has been gross recession of alveolar bone or flaps have been raised past the reflection of the mucous membrane. A finger should be placed at once below the root and kept there to prevent it going deeper. A flap may be raised to expose the root which can then be lifted out using a blunt hooked instrument. Attempts should not be made to grasp it with forceps as if they fail to grip the root they may drive it deeper into the space.

The tissue spaces. In the mandible, roots or teeth can be lost in the tissue spaces of the floor of the mouth either above or below the mylohyoid muscle. The lower third molar roots can be pushed down lingually through the bottom of the socket if this is deficient, as does occasionally occur; the root then lies below the mylohyoid. During the extraction of the unerupted lower third molar it can be elevated lingually into the tissue spaces. In all these cases the grave danger is that the tooth will pass into the deeper planes of the neck as a result of gravity and movements of the muscles. Without delay a finger must be placed either extra- or intraorally to stop the tooth moving. A flap may then be raised to explore the tissue space when the tooth may be 'milked' out or removed as described for those under the periosteum. When the tooth is lying superficial to the mylohyoid removal is better delayed to allow an extraoral approach, followed by a blunt dissection up to the tooth.

The unerupted upper third molar can be elevated distally into the soft tissue space behind the tuberosity of the maxilla to lie in the pterygomandibular space. This is explored through an incision made down the anterior border of the ascending ramus of the mandible.

Bone cavities. The roots of the maxillary second premolar, first, second and third molars and occasionally the first premolar are related to the maxillary sinus into which they can be displaced during extraction. Unerupted and supernumerary teeth may be related to the floor of the nose. Lower apices can be pushed into the inferior dental canal. In both jaws roots can be driven into pathological cavities such as cysts or abscesses. Where it is suspected that a root is lost in a bone cavity the operation is stopped and radiographs are taken in two planes at right angles to each other in an effort to localise the lost root or tooth.

Roots displaced into the inferior dental canal are removed by a transalveolar approach, care being taken not to damage the inferior dental nerve. They should not be left as they may give rise to infection or pressure symptoms of paraesthesia or anaesthesia. Roots pushed into the nose, if they lie under the mucous membrane, are usually easily recovered through the socket, or through the anterior nares if they are lying in the nasal cavity.

Oro-antral fistula and root in antrum

Oro-antral fistula

The relationship of the apices of the maxillary premolar and molar teeth to the maxillary sinus is variable and depends on individual anatomy and the age of the patient as pneumatisation of the sinus continues throughout life. Often the antrum dips down between the roots of the molar teeth which virtually form part of the antral floor.

Occasionally the uncomplicated extraction of a tooth may fracture the thin floor of the sinus and cause an oroantral communication. Apical infection can destroy the bone over the apex, bringing an apical granuloma into contact with antral lining which is then torn by the extraction of the tooth. Infection in the maxillary sinus may also predispose to the establishment of a fistula. More commonly the communication is produced by attempts to remove retained apices so that the antrum floor is perforated or the apex displaced into it.

Signs and symptoms. The patient will complain of air passing from the nose into the mouth and this the operator will be able to see bubbling through the communication, particularly when the patient is asked to breathe out. Blood from the wound and mouthwashes used to rinse the mouth may pass through the sinus into the nose. A blunt probe passed very gently into the socket will be found to penetrate into the maxillary sinus. This last test should rarely be performed as it may create a communication. Established fistulae tend to reduce in diameter but the track from mouth to sinus frequently fails to heal spontaneously and becomes epithelialised. When this is large the patient complains that drinks pass from the mouth into the nose, that cigarettes are inhaled with difficulty, and that air passes into the mouth. As the hole shrinks it remains a pathway for infection, but fails to provide adequate drainage for the sinus so that often the symptoms of acute sinusitis are superimposed on those of those of a fistula.

Treatment. Immediately the surgeon finds he has created a communication he should check that the tooth has been completely extracted. He should then gently remove all pieces of loose bone that might form sequestra. The buccal plate of alveolar bone is trimmed if a flap has been raised, but is otherwise left alone. Irrigation is best avoided. The mucous membrane over the socket is gently drawn together with simple interrupted sutures and every effort made to obtain a sound clot in the socket. *Under no circumstances should the socket be packed.* Impressions are taken and a splint constructed with a flange to cover and protect the socket. Before taking the impressions a sizeable piece of foil should be placed over the socket to protect the clot and to prevent the impression material being forced into the communication. The splint should be produced quickly as an emergency measure and, if possible, put in place the same day. Antibiotic therapy is commenced immediately and continued for some five days as a prophylactic measure whether or not there is a history of previous sinusitis. The patient is instructed that under no circumstances must he raise the pressure in his nose by blowing it until healing has taken place. Such energetic measures immediately applied will in most cases result in satisfactory healing by first intention.

Where the above measures fail and the fistula remains patent after six weeks, but there are no signs of maxillary sinus infection, a surgical repair should be undertaken without delay. This may be done under general anaesthesia as an in-patient or local anaesthesia as an out-patient, but always under an antibiotic cover started one hour before operation. There are two satisfactory methods, one using a buccal and the other a palatal flap to cover the defect. In both cases the operation commences by excising the fistula cleanly and curetting out the tract from the socket. The deeper

Fig. 45 Left section shows maxillary sinus together with the second premolar tooth socket and small apical cystic area in contact with the antral floor. Right section of same subject shows nasal wall with conchae removed.

Transverse lines pass through both sections at the same levels: upper line through the ostium of the maxillary sinus; middle line along the floor of the nose at the level of the inferior meatus; lower line at the apices of the premolar teeth. These stress the inadequacy of the natural drainage in infection.

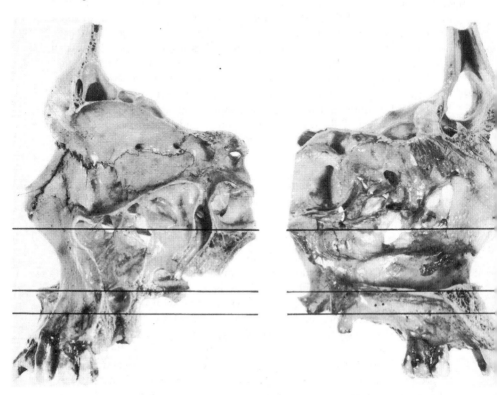

part of the fistula adjoining the antrum may be left undisturbed where there is no evidence of infection.

Buccal flap. This is the operation of choice. The flap is raised by making an incision along the buccal edge of the socket concerned and two vertical incisions from the cervical margins of the adjacent teeth obliquely up into the buccal sulcus. The flap is carefully raised well past the reflection. Normally this would not cover the socket because the periosteum is still attached, beyond the reflection, to maxillary bone. To overcome this the periosteum *only* is divided by a long horizontal incision made well *above* the line of reflection of the mucosa. It will then be found that the flap can be drawn down over the socket without tension (Fig. 46). Buttonholing of the buccal flap must obviously be avoided. The palatal mucoperiosteum is then trimmed back to a straight line so that the line of closure will be supported by palatal bone. This margin is raised slightly to permit eversion

Fig. 46 Closure of oroantral fistula using a buccal flap. (*a*) Show excision of fistula and buccal incision through mucoperiosteum. (*b*) Flap raised; note palatal mucosa trimmed back to expose ledge of palatal bone. (*c*) Dotted line shows incision through *periosteum only* above line of reflection of mucosa. (*d*) Mucosa extended once periosteum is divided. (*e*) and (*f*) Closure effected with buccal flap resting on palatal bone.

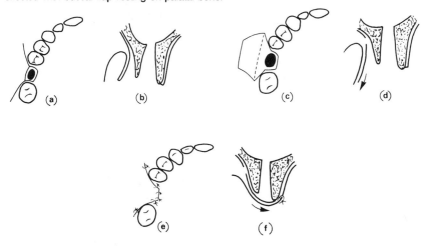

of its edges when suturing. Haemorrhage is carefully arrested as a haematoma could prevent the flap taking, and closure is effected with mattress sutures. A splint may be worn over the wound to protect it. The only disadvantage of this operation is that it may reduce the depth of the buccal sulcus opposite the socket concerned.

Palatal flap. The palatal flap is a pedicle flap which derives its blood supply from the palatine artery and therefore has its base over the greater palatine foramen. It is raised by making an incision in the palate parallel to the cervical margins of the teeth but about 5 mm above them. This extends from the second molar to the lateral incisor and is then taken back almost down the midline of the palate. The flap is carefully raised with the periosteum to include the palatine artery. This must be preserved because if its function is impaired the flap will be deprived of its blood supply and die (Fig. 47). A second hazard to the artery occurs when the flap is rotated to cover the fistula, because if it is twisted too sharply, the blood supply may be cut off. Indeed this fact limits its use to the second premolar and first molar sockets. The buccal flap is trimmed back to a clean edge and, if possible, supported on bone though often loss of the buccal alveolar plate at the time of extraction makes this difficult to achieve. The flap is sutured into place with mattress sutures and the bone deficiency in the palate covered with a dressing (Fig. 47b). It has the advantage that the palatal flap is very thick and tough and is of sufficient length to cover the whole socket.

Infected maxillary sinus. Where the maxillary sinus is infected closure must not be attempted until this has settled.

Fig. 47 Oroantral fistula. (a) design of palatal flap for closure of fistula showing the palatine artery in the flap and the excision of the fistula. (b) Closure showing rotation of the palatal flap and pack sutured over the area of bare bone.

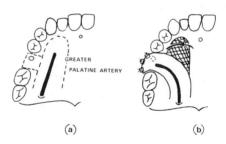

(a)   (b)

Acute sinusitis. In acute sinusitis the patient complains of pain together with a feeling of weight in the cheek on the affected side, especially on bending down. Discharge from the maxillary sinus is often described as 'catarrh' on that side, especially in the morning. Examination often shows the cheek over the infected sinus to be red, there is tenderness on pressure in the canine fossa and pus may be seen and smelled in the nostril. Transillumination and radiographs show opacity and, if pus is present, a fluid level (Fig. 48). Careful examination of the fistula will often show it to be inflamed or filled with granulations and discharging pus. The acute phase is treated with antibacterial drugs, and ephedrine nasal drops to reduce nasal congestion, and improve drainage through the ostium. Where this proves inadequate the advice of an otorhinolaryngologist is required as intranasal antrostomy in the inferior meatus (Fig. 45) may be necessary to improve drainage. Washing out the sinuses is contraindicated in the acute phase but may be performed for a chronic infection. Gentle irrigation is used either through the fistula or an antrostomy with warm normal saline every three days until the washings are clear. At this stage closure of the fistula may be completed provided that satisfactory drainage for the antrum into the nose is present.

Root in antrum

When a root is believed to have been pushed into the maxillary sinus the surgeon should first examine the socket carefully, and the adjacent sockets, lest it should have been displaced there. He then considers whether the root is lying below the antral lining or has penetrated it to enter the sinus. Presence of an oro-antral fistula is strong, but not conclusive, evidence that the root is in the antrum. Radiographs, apical intraoral and oblique occlusal films are required (Fig. 49). It is usual to take a second set after shaking the head to see if the root has moved, if it has it is probably lying free in the sinus cavity. The root if fixed may be jammed under the lining, though this is not certain as it can be lying in the antrum anchored by a blood clot.

Fig. 48 Occipito-mental radiograph of fluid level in right antrum.

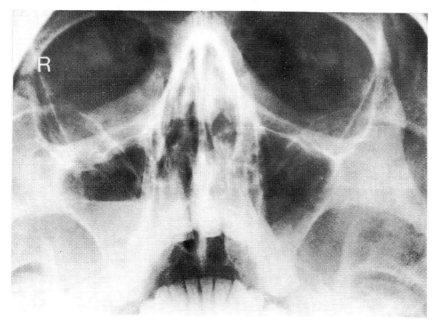

Where the root is believed to be lying under the lining it may be removed through a transalveolar approach, care being taken not to damage the antral lining. This is better than through an extranasal antrostomy as it is often very difficult to locate roots under the lining when looking into the antrum.

Fig. 49 Radiograph of root displaced into the antrum.

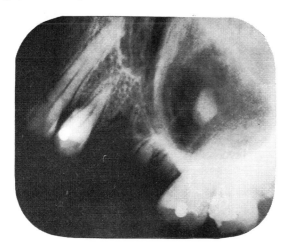

Roots which are lying in the antral cavity and remain in close relation to the socket are best removed through a transalveolar approach. Where the root is grossly displaced the Caldwell–Luc extranasal antrostomy is preferable. For this latter operation the patient is admitted to hospital and, under general anaesthesia and an antibiotic cover, an incision is made in the mucous membrane of the canine fossa above its reflection into the cheek. A flap is reflected to expose the anterior wall of the antrum. The infraorbital nerve must not be damaged, particularly by stretching when retracting the flap during the operation. With chisels or burs a round hole about 1.5 cm in diameter is cut through the thin anterior wall, above the roots of the teeth and near to the lateral wall of the nose. All spicules of loose bone are carefully removed and the interior inspected using a headlamp. Suction should be used very carefully to avoid damaging the delicate lining. The root is lifted out with sinus forceps and, if infection is present, drainage is provided by a tube drain inserted through the buccal incision. The mouth wound is then closed.

Damage to soft tissues

The chief cause is carelessness by the operator. The gingivae can be torn by misapplication of dental forceps, pulling on teeth to which gingival margins are still attached instead of dissecting them free, and by attempting the removal of roots without adequate access. When extracting upper teeth the lower lip can be trapped between the forceps and the lower teeth.

The cheek, tongue, floor of mouth and palate can be damaged by instruments which slip because they are not properly supported. This applies particularly to elevators, burs and discs. A disc guard must always be used. Burns are caused by hot instruments from the steriliser, overheating of burs or handpieces, and antiseptic solutions.

Nerves. The inferior dental nerve can be damaged during the extraction of buried teeth or retained roots. Its relationship to the third molar has been discussed (Chapter IX). When a flap is raised for operations in the lower premolar area the mental nerve should be identified and preserved. Stretching of nerves when retracting flaps can produce paraesthesia which may be very painful and of long duration and this can occur with the mental and infraorbital nerves. The lingual nerve where it lies in the lingual mucoperiosteum of the mandible opposite the third molar can be damaged when this tooth is being extracted.

Fracture of alveolar and basal bone

The buccal and lingual alveolar plates. These can be fractured during the extraction of teeth, particularly if as a result of chronic periodontal disease the tooth is ankylosed or exostosed to the socket wall. The buccal plate in the molar region is most frequently involved but is usually firmly attached to periosteum which provides it with a satisfactory blood supply. This bone can be retained if it is repositioned by gently compressing the socket between finger and thumb after completing the extractions.

Loose fragments not attached to periosteum must be removed lest they form sequestra, suppurate and delay healing.

Occasionally extraction of a tooth causes a horizontal fracture of the alveolus which may carry other teeth. This occurs classically in the maxilla during an attempted extraction of single standing upper molars, especially the third molar, and may cause fracture of the tuberosity. This will be felt during the extraction by the movement of bone rather than the tooth and a radiograph should be taken to confirm the presence of a fracture. Where the portion of bone attached to the tooth is small, bone and tooth should be dissected out by blunt dissection through a buccal flap, taking every precaution to prevent tearing of the mucous membrane. The antrum is frequently opened following this manoeuvre, but if the flaps are healthy it can be closed satisfactorily. The surgeon may wish to retain a large piece of bone or one with other teeth, not for extraction, attached to it. It is very difficult to hold the bone still and complete the planned extraction. So long as any pain from the tooth can be alleviated the fragment can be splinted for a month until it is firm. The tooth may then be extracted by freeing it from the bone with burs and gently prising it out with elevators. This procedure is seldom justified unless sound teeth in occlusion are to be saved.

Basal bone. The predisposing causes of fracture of the body of the mandible are general bone diseases (osteogenesis imperfecta, osteopetrosis), weakened bone owing to age, osteomyelitis, cysts, tumours, teeth with large or misplaced roots and buried teeth. The immediate cause is misapplication of instruments or the use of undue force, particularly with elevators. As soon as the operator realises that a fracture has occurred he should complete the operation if this can be done without causing further damage. Radiographs must be taken to confirm the position and extent of the injury, and the patient referred immediately for treatment by reduction and fixation (Chapter XIV).

Dislocation of the temporomandibular joint

This occurs most frequently following the extraction of lower teeth under general anaesthesia but may happen even under local anaesthesia in those patients who have a lax capsule and weak supporting muscles.

Dislocation may be prevented by supporting the mandible firmly and never exerting more force in the primary downward movement than can be opposed by the supporting hand. During extractions under local anaesthesia a prop placed on the opposite side of the mouth gives the patient something to bite on and thereby support his jaw.

At the close of operations under general anaesthesia the jaws should be brought together with the teeth in occlusion at the time the prop and pack are removed from the mouth. The jaw, if dislocated, may be reduced before the patient returns to full consciousness (Chapter XVII).

Haemorrhage

Prolonged haemorrhage is a common complication following extraction of teeth and occurs as primary (Chapter VII), reactionary and secondary haemorhage. The most important aspect of treatment is pevention. The systemic causes have been discussed in Chapter III, but local factors are more often responsible for post-operative haemorrhage. These include infection, excessive trauma and local vascular lesions.

Infections include gingival conditions, which should be treated by scaling and instructions in oral hygiene. To be effective scaling should be completed a week before operation and mouth-brushing conscientiously undertaken by the patient. This preparation should be done for all but emergency extractions, and the dental surgeon must stress the importance of a clean mouth as many patients tend to neglect oral hygiene on the ground that they are about to lose their remaining teeth. Where there is an apical or pericoronal condition the use of antibiotics may be indicated, not only to prevent a flare up but to protect the blood clot from destruction by bacteria.

Reactionary haemorrhage. This occurs within forty-eight hours of the operation or accident when a local rise in blood pressure may force open divided vessels insecurely sealed by natural or artificial means. It is common in patients recovering from shock and in those treated under local anaesthesia when the effect of the vasoconstrictor wears off. It is arrested by one of the methods described below and, for excited patients, by administration of a sedative.

Secondary haemorrhage. The cause of this is infection which destroys the blood clot or may ulcerate a vessel wall. It starts about seven days after operation usually with a mild ooze which is a serious symptom in wounds near major vessels because, if the vessel is not found and ligated, a massive haemorrhage may ensue. In the more mild capillary form such as from a tooth socket it will be more troublesome than dangerous. Bleeding is arrested by local measures and antibacterial drugs are prescribed to combat the infection.

Treatment. A practitioner who is called to a post-extraction haemorrhage should first take from the patient, or a relative, a *rapid* history which must include the number of teeth extracted, the duration of bleeding (the volume of the loss is unreliable as it is invariably diluted by saliva), and whether there has been any similar previous occurrence or known blood dyscrasia. The patient's general condition is then rapidly assessed and, if he appears shocked and ill, arrangements must be made at once for transfer to hospital. Meanwhile the dental surgeon will apply local measures to arrest the bleeding.

It is never a waste of time to clean the patient, for much of the distress and fear associated with bleeding is due to the sight of blood on the face, sheets and clothes. The mouth is then examined in a good light with adequate suction apparatus, if available. The latter should only be used to remove blood from the floor of the mouth and not be applied to the sockets since aspiration will disturb stable blood clots and encourage further bleeding. Pressure is then applied by placing a finger on each side of the alveolus to find the bleeding point. If this is successful in arresting the haemorrhage it indicates bleeding from soft tissues, and sutures may be placed across the socket. Where pressure fails to arrest the haemorrhage, bleeding is from the bony socket and a Whitehead's varnish pack may be placed in the socket. When local measures have controlled the bleeding, the patient's general condition should be more accurately assessed by recording his pulse and blood pressure. He should receive supportive treatment including warmth, administration of fluids by mouth, and drugs to relieve anxiety and pain.

Surgical emphysema

This is a collection of air which has been forced into the tissue spaces through the extraction wound and forms a swelling which characteristically crackles on palpation. It results from increased air pressure in the mouth from using an air spray, or blowing a trumpet or a balloon. Surgical emphysema seldom gives rise to discomfort, but settles without treatment as the air is slowly absorbed.

Delay healing and infection

Normally a tooth socket heals by second intention, the blood clot becoming organised as capillaries and fibroblasts grow into it from the bony or soft tissue periphery. The blood clot may fail to form if there is little bleeding owing to sclerosis of the bone forming the tooth socket, the action of the vasoconstrictor present in the local anaesthetic solution, or packing of the socket to arrest haemorrhage. Infection may rapidly supervene if the extracted tooth was septic or contamination takes place from the mouth. Even where a satisfactory clot does form, this can be destroyed by bacteria either present in the socket or introduced by imperfectly sterilised instruments. Lacerated or bruised tissues, loose pieces of bone, or retained tooth fragments also favour secondary infection.

A septic socket is typically inflamed at the gum margins and either contains the remains of the blood clot or is filled with food debris. It is very painful. Because of its appearance, clinicians call it a 'dry socket', a misnomer that fails to stress the importance of infection in its aetiology.

Where no clot forms at the time of operation recourse is made to packing the socket loosely with ribbon gauze impregnated with Whitehead's varnish. The treatment of established septic sockets is directed to the control of pain by the use of analgesics, to irrigation with warm physiological saline to remove food debris, and to dressing the cavity to protect it from further contamination and painful stimuli. Packing with bismuth, iodoform, paraffin paste (B.I.P.P.) and lignocaine paste on ribbon gauze very effectively protects the socket and settles the acute pain. The dressings are not changed too frequently, the first after two days and thereafter each week until the socket is epithelialised. Other authorities prefer zinc oxide and eugenol packs which, though effective, unfortunately set hard and can be difficult and painful to remove. Hot salt water mouth baths held over the socket should be used every hour for two or three days.

Post-extraction infection may take another form in which exuberant granulations and a discharge of pus localised to the socket appear a week or so after the extraction. Frequently bone sequestra are the cause and when they are removed healing takes place rapidly. This condition is relatively painless and the granulations make packing difficult. Treatment is first by hot mouth baths but, if these fail to settle the socket, radiographs are necessary to confirm the local nature of the infection. The socket is then opened up, sequestra and granulations removed and the cavity packed open. Forceful curettage is contraindicated as it may spread the infection.

Infected sockets are a serious condition which if neglected may progress to osteomyelitis or to a severe cellulitis of the face and neck. (Chapter XII).

Damage to other organs

Faulty or careless handling of instruments may result in damage to other organs. Under general anaesthesia the eyes, if not suitably protected, can be damaged by caustic fluids, instruments and the operator's fingers.

Pain

Post-extraction pain may result from incomplete extraction of the tooth, laceration of the soft tissues, exposed bone, infected sockets or damage to adjacent nerves. Treatment is by eliminating the cause and symptomatic by prescribing analgesic drugs.

Swelling

Swelling or oedema following surgery is part of the inflammatory reaction to surgical interference. It is increased by a poor surgical technique, particularly rough handling of the tissues, pulling on flaps to gain access and inadequate drainage. There is also a wide individual variation in the response to trauma which does not seem to be related to any of these factors.

Trismus

This may occur as the result of oedema and swelling, in which case opening improves as the swelling resolves. Damage to the temporomandibular joint due to excessive downward pressure or to keeping the patient's mouth open wide for a long period of time may lead to a more chronic, painful condition with symptoms of the pain dysfunction syndrome (Chapter XVII). The injection for the inferior dental nerve block may cause a painless trismus without swelling which has variously been ascribed to trauma to the medial pterygoid muscle causing spasm, or to penetration of a small blood vessel and formation of a haematoma. As the haematoma organises so the trismus becomes apparent, often starting two to three days after the injection. It will recover with time, usually six weeks, but may be improved more quickly by gently opening the mouth under a general anaesthetic.

Broken instruments

All instruments should be carefully examined after use and any that are defective immediately discarded or sent for repair. Should one break, a search is made at once for the fragment and if it is not recovered radiographs are taken to locate it. If the instrument is sterile and the piece small, such as the point of a suture needle or a tiny portion of a dental bur, this may be left and the patient informed.

Broken local anaesthetic needles occur chiefly when giving an inferior dental nerve block. The needle should never be inserted up to the hub but one-third of its length must be kept clear of the tissues. A pair of artery forceps should always be close at hand to grasp the fragment immediately before it disappears if the patient moves or swallows.

Removal of broken needles from the pterygomandibular space is a difficult operation. First the needle must be localised by taking radiographs in two planes (lateral oblique and posterior anterior views of the mandible), preferably with a second needle in position to serve as a marker. At operation, performed under endotracheal anaesthesia, a vertical incision is made parallel to the anterior border of the ascending ramus and blunt dissection is performed down to the marker and a search is made in the vicinity for the broken needle. A metallic foreign body detector can be of great assistance.

Mishaps

The patient or a relative should always be warned beforehand if any serious difficulty or complication is envisaged and this should be entered on the consent form signed by the patient.

When a mishap has occurred it is important to keep quite calm and not become emotionally involved. The patient is often upset, aggressive and vociferous, and the surgeon must not allow himself to get caught up in this mood. He may, and indeed should, state what has happened quite factually without making any comment or explanation which might imply liability. If the patient is nervous it is best to tell a sensible relative or, failing that, the patient's medical or dental practitioner. In any serious accident, such as a fracture of the jaw or a root in antrum, it is very wise to hand the case over to a colleague, preferably a specialist, as thereafter the responsibility is shared. It is also wise when treating a mishap to limit the immediate care to putting it right, and not to attempt the completion of all the surgery planned, as a new disaster may occur elsewhere in the mouth.

In any case of doubt the practitioners' protection society should be informed at the earliest possible time and asked for advice and guidance, which they will willingly give.

Further reading

Killey, H. C. and Kay, L. W. (1977), *The Prevention of Complications in Dental Surgery*, 2nd edn. Churchill Livingstone, Edinburgh.

Robinson, P. P. (1988), 'Observations on the recovery of sensation following inferior alveolar nerve injuries', *Brit. J. O. M. Surg.*, **26**, 177.

XI Preparation of the mouth for dentures

The surgical preparation of the mouth for dentures begins at the time the first permanent tooth is extracted. At this and all subsequent operations the dental surgeon must try to leave a satisfactory base to support a prosthesis and he should consider the form the denture-bearing tissues will present when healing and resorption of bone is complete. Edentulous patients should not be subjected to surgery to improve the stability, comfort or aesthetic appearance of their dentures without the opinion of a specialist prosthetist.

Ideally, treatment for those undergoing clearances or surgical preparation for dentures should be planned jointly. This assists the surgeon and enables the prosthetist to make valuable pre-operative records of the occlusion and of the tooth form and shade. Further, to assist denture retention certain teeth may be selected for conservation rather than extraction. Consideration should be given to retaining roots and provision of overdentures to maintain alveolar bone height. In general dental practice, surgeon and prosthetist are one and the same person, offering an unrivalled opportunity for treatment planning and for long-term evaluation of the results of surgery. The oral surgeon will learn much from reviewing his patients over several years and discussing, with the dental surgeon who constructs the denture, any problems that occur.

Preservation of alveolar bone

It should always be borne in mind that alveolar bone is precious and once lost cannot be replaced. This tissue, possibly more than any other, suffers from instrument mismanagement. A conservative approach and a careful surgical technique will help to reduce prosthetic difficulties later.

During extractions the alveolar bone may be damaged or fractured by the use of excessive force or worse, by the inclusion of the socket wall within the forcep blades. The commonest site of alveolar fracture is the buccal plate opposite the upper molars. This, if still attached to periosteum, may be preserved and pressed back into place, but if detached from its blood supply it should be removed to avoid sequestration and delayed healing. Fracture and loss of the maxillary tuberosity may interfere with retention of the upper denture by making the peripheral seal at this point inadequate.

The bone of the edentulous jaws in the elderly is often dense and brittle whilst resorption of the alveolar ridge has made it less strong. Under such conditions the extraction of buried teeth and roots is difficult. Those that are symptomless need not be extracted if they are covered by bone and are unlikely to come to the surface during the life of the denture. Those lying superficially or associated with secondary disease such as cysts or granulomas should be removed. Roots and teeth must be accurately localised and tooth division practised to reduce the amount of bone removed. This is confined as far as possible to the buccal aspect and osteoplastic flaps are used to preserve the ridge where teeth are lying in it (Chapter IX).

The use of blunt burs or failure to provide irrigation with a continuous stream of saline can cause overheating with subsequent necrosis of bone.

Surgical preparation at the time of extraction of teeth

The operation is carefully planned to include the removal of buried teeth, roots, or other lesions. Any necessary adjustments to the alveolar bone are marked on plaster models and, because this bone can never be replaced, every effort is made to reduce cutting or smoothing to a minimum. Difficult extractions are best completed through a planned transalveolar approach to avoid accidental alveolar fractures which lead to widespread trimming to produce an acceptable ridge. For multirooted teeth, particularly upper molars, division of the roots so that each is removed separately may conserve alveolar bone. Access to deeply buried roots or teeth can often be made through the lateral aspect of the alveolus, to leave the ridge intact. In all such operations bone cutting should be limited to one side, leaving the lingual or palatal plate and its mucoperiosteum untouched. Alveolectomy at the time of extraction requires careful consideration as, even after radical surgical reduction, some natural resorption takes place and it is impossible to tell how extensive this will be. Generally it is advisable to do the minimum at the time of extraction and wait for at least three months to reconsider the situation when healing and natural remodelling has taken place. A conservative approach is important where periodontal disease has already caused appreciable bone loss.

There are certain indications for minor surgery at the time of the extractions.

First jagged or irregular alveolar margins and septal bone: these are treated by dividing the buccal interdental papillae from the lingual along the ridge and exposing the bony edges of the sockets just enough to smooth the bone with a bur or file, after which the mucosa is closed over the ridge.

Second, minor local deformities, such as fibrous bands, bulbous tuberosities, and undercuts may be removed.

Third the premaxilla may need reduction in cases of superior protrusion.

Surgery for immediate restoration dentures

Where a complete immediate denture is to be provided the posterior teeth are first extracted. Sufficient teeth are left in the premolar region to maintain the vertical dimension of the occlusion while the sockets are healing. Three months later the rest of the teeth are removed. When, owing to the tightness of the lip, an anterior flange cannot be worn an open-faced denture with the anterior teeth socketed into the alveolus is provided as a temporary measure until natural resorption has taken place. In certain cases, however, it is obvious that some reduction is necessary at the time the teeth are extracted.

Where the patient must be admitted to hospital the less satisfactory procedure of fitting a full mouth immediate restoration denture can be performed.

Alveolectomy for pre-maxillary protrusion. The prosthetist and the surgeon who is to do the operation should examine the patient and prepare the models for the dentures. Articulated models in duplicate and panoramic radiographs are required. On one model the teeth on one side only are removed and the plaster trimmed back to a satisfactory depth, which must not be more than half the diameter of the sockets (Fig. 50), and teeth are set up to occlude with the lower dentition to estimate the improvement achieved.

Fig. 50 Trimming of models for alveolectomy. *Above left:* preoperative models articulated to show maxillary protrusion. *Above right:* Duplicate maxillary model with one half trimmed, used for comparison and reference. *Below left:* Completely trimmed original model with template in place. *Below right:* Duplicate model with teeth set up on patient's left only, to show improvement achieved.

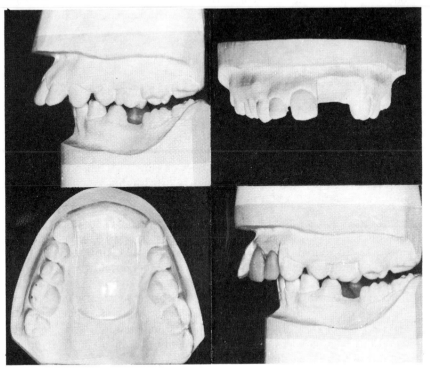

Frequently it will be necessary to reduce the height of the alveolus to give sufficient space to fit artificial teeth. When one half of the model is prepared the untouched half provides a useful comparative record of the original state. The second model is then trimmed to the same amount but on both sides and used to process the dentures. A thin template in clear acrylic, which must be quite transparent, is prepared on a duplicate of this model.

At operation an incision is made round the necks of the teeth with two short vertical extensions just beyond the standing teeth at each end. The teeth are then extracted and the flap reflected. Using rongeurs or a large rosehead bur, the ridge is cut to the size planned and left smooth with no sharp projections from the interradicular septa. The soft tissues are then replaced and the transparent template pressed firmly over them. High spots show as blanched areas of mucous membrane. These need further reduction before final smoothing is completed with a bone file.

Surgical preparation of the edentulous mouth

Before prosthetic surgery the edentulous patient must have a clinical examination and panoramic radiographs to avoid missing conditions such as buried roots or residual cysts. The surgery requires skill and patience as the soft tissues can be difficult to manipulate and slow to heal owing to scarring following repeated ulceration or to friability caused by the atrophic changes of age. The operation must leave minimal scarring so placed that it receives the least pressure from the dentures.

Bony irregularities

Torus. A large palatal torus is usually acceptable if smooth but when nodular or irregular in shape may need to be removed. Tori, often bilateral, are sometimes found on the lingual aspect of the mandible in the premolar region and can cause pain or difficulty when a full denture is worn. The torus palatinus is excised through a Y-shaped midline sagittal incision and the bony prominence removed with burs or chisels. A full denture lined with a periodontal dressing is immediately fitted to hold the flap in place and prevent formation of a haematoma.

Alveolar ridges. These should be of substantial size, as the greater their surface area the better is the denture retained and the more evenly are masticatory pressures distributed. In grossly resorbed ridges the dentures are loose as there is nothing to resist horizontal displacement. This may be aggrevated by failure of the peripheral seal due to the lifting action of certain muscles (buccinator, mylohyoid and genioglossus) the attachments of which become level with the alveolar crest. In the mandible the mental foramen can open on the crest of the ridge and cause pain from pressure of the denture. Occasionally ridges may be too high making it difficult to fit dentures without over opening the vertical dimension.

Undercut ridges are unfavourable if the flange has to be built out from the alveolus to avoid them as this reduces the peripheral seal. However, certain undercuts may be retained to assist retention providing the problem of fitting the denture round them can be overcome.

Even when considerable resorption of the edentulous ridge has taken place it may be irregular. This can follow tooth extraction where the expanded buccal plate has not been adequately compressed or when it fractures and jagged edges are left. These cause pain when the mucosa is compressed between the sharp bone and the denture during chewing.

Alveolectomy. This is the operation used to smooth irregular ridges and remove undercuts. Radiographs must be studied to determine the extent of the antrum and the position of the mental nerve. Plaster casts of the ridges are used to assist planning so that the procedure is completed with the least destruction of alveolar bone.

A horizontal incision is made on the buccal aspect of the alveolus through fixed mucoperiosteum just short of non-keratinised mucosa so that this is not disturbed by the operation. Two veretical incisions are taken over the crest of the alveolus and on to the lingual or palatal mucosa. The flap is reflected to expose the alveolar crest (Fig. 51). The bone may be trimmed with a large rosehead bur or rongeurs and smoothed with a bone file. The operator then replaces the flap and runs his finger over the ridge to check it is smooth. The wound is thoroughly irrigated with saline and if much reduction has taken place the flap is trimmed conservatively. The wound is closed without tension on the mucoperiosteum.

Feather edge ridge. This condition occurs in the lower anterior region beneath a full lower denture. The patient complains of inability to wear the denture for more than one or two hours owing to soreness. The ridge is usually very narrow and covered with thin atrophic mucosa which is inflamed and tender to palpation. Radiographs show an uneven resorbed ridge which has no cortical plate but a feathered appearance due to spicules of bone standing vertically (Fig. 52).

Fig. 51 Alveolectomy. *B* indicates buccal aspect of ridge. (*a*) Arrow shows level of buccal horizontal incision above the reflection. (*b*) Flap raised from buccal to lingual to expose alveolar ridge without interference with attachment of mucoperiosteum at the buccal or lingual reflection.

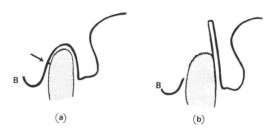

(a)　　　　　(b)

Fig. 52 Radiograph showing feather-edged ridge.

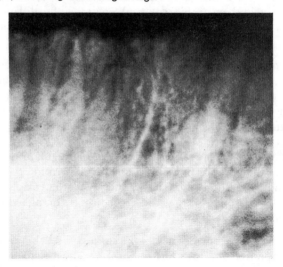

Surgery should be considered only when all prosthetic techniques to reduce the load (selective compression impressions, narrow teeth and resilient linings) have failed.

Treatment. Surgical treatment has not proved to be very effective. Alveolectomy may be performed but when this is limited to smoothing the knife-edge ridge relief is usually only temporary. Even when the ridge is drastically reduced, so that the denture virtually rests on basal bone, the symptoms often persist. In view of this, attention has been directed to the mucosa. Though histological examination has shown scant changes in this, better results have been obtained by excising the mucoperiosteum over the ridge and replacing it with a free mucoperiosteal graft taken from the maxillary ridge or palate.

Genial tubercles. These sometimes become prominent in the floor of the mouth owing to alveolar recession. They are best left, as genioglossus is attached to them. Occasionally, the upper part of a prominent genial tubercule may require excision to facilitate denture wearing.

Mylohyoid ridge removal. Where the mandibular alveolus has undergone gross resorption the mylohyoid ridge, if sharp, may be a source of pain under the lower denture. Its removal, by cutting off the attachment of the mylohyoid muscle, does deepen the lingual sulcus of the mandible and may assist denture retention when the muscle attachment is level with the alveolar crest.

An incision is made along the alveolar crest and reflected lingually to expose the mylohyoid muscle which is detached from the bone. The prominent bony mylohyoid ridge is then separated from the mandible with burs or chisels. Bleeding is meticulously arrested and the incision closed. This procedure may be carried out in combination with sulcus deepening in the anterior mandible (see p. 137).

Soft tissue irregularities

Flabby ridges. Ideally the alveolar mucosa should be firm and closely adherent to the ridge, but after the extraction of teeth for periodontal disease hyperplastic tissue may remain to form a flabby ridge. More often such ridges are found in the anterior region of the maxilla when a full upper denture is opposed only by the natural lower anterior teeth. The excessive pressure causes resorption of the maxillary bone leaving a thick mobile fibrous ridge offering an unstable support for the denture. However, as this is better than the completely flat surface often left by surgery, the prosthetist prefers to manage this problem with special impression techniques and denture design. An alternative approach is to augment the underlying bone using a bone substitute material to provide support for the soft tissue.

Reduction of tuberosities. Large maxillary tuberosities with deep sulci assist denture retention but if too large they encroach on the space available for dentures. Many have appreciable bony undercuts on their buccal aspect which, if unilateral, can be used to improve denture stability but when present bilaterally prevent a satisfactory fit. Radiographs before surgery are necessary to identify unerupted upper third molars, to establish the relationship between soft tissue and alveolar bone and to determine the extent of the maxillary antrum.

Treatment. A fibrous tuberosity may be reduced by making palatal and buccal incisions down to bone to excise an ellipse of mucous membrane, fibrous tissue and periosteum from the crest of the ridge. To facilitate closure the incisions are carried forward to meet in the first molar region. The raw

Fig. 53 Reduction of the tuberosity. (a) *Above:* Elliptical incision over tuberosity. *Below:* Cross-section of excision showing deep portion secondarily excised (shaded) to allow flaps to be apposed on bone without tension. (*b*) Closure.

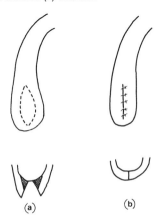

(a)   (b)

edges are then undermined and the underlying fibrous tissue removed to produce a reduction in the height of the ridge and to allow satisfactory closure (Fig. 53). The space between upper and lower ridges is checked to be satisfactory before the wound is sutured.

Where only the bone is to be reduced in height or a buccal undercut removed the approach is made through an alveolectomy flap. Care is required not to perforate the antral lining when cutting bone in this region. Usually both bone and soft tissue are to be reduced and the elliptical incision is used to expose the ridge by reflecting the edges of the wound. Buccal undercuts in this area are often found high above the crest making a vertical incision at the anterior buccal edge of the ellipse necessary.

Fraenectomy. A fraenum is a musculo-fibrous band attached to the alveolus and inserted into the muscles of the face. The most important of these are the labial fraena in the mid-line of the upper and lower jaw, the buccal fraena in the premolar region and the lingual fraenum of the mandible. During movements of the facial muscles they lift the dentures and so break the peripheral seal. The denture can usually be relieved round them but where the ridges have resorbed this may greatly reduce the possible depth of the flange and even weaken the denture, making surgery by excision necessary.

Treatment. The maxillary labial fraenum is excised as follows. First the extent of its attachment to the maxilla is found by drawing the upper lip forward to put the fraenum on tension. This causes the base to blanch and it is frequently seen to extend palatally into the incisive papilla. The whole length of the fraenum and the mucosa over it is removed but the periosteum is left intact. A diamond-shaped incision is made round the margins of the band sufficiently deep to allow it to be dissected out and for the portion in the lip to be superficially exicsed (Fig. 54). The mucosa is undermined before suturing. The effect of suturing the lateral edges of the diamond-shaped incision together is to lengthen the wound and mobilise the soft tissues. This allows a greater depth of sulcus to be achieved.

Fraena may be lengthened by making a *horizontal* incision across the middle of the band which passes through the *whole depth* of the fibrous tissue it contains. The mucosal edges are undermined and the incision is sutured *vertically* (Fig. 54b).

Fig. 54 Fraena. (*a*) Incision for excision of labial fraenum. (*b*) Lingual fraenum lengthened by making a horizontal incison *A–B* and suturing it vertically.

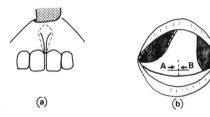

Denture irritation hyperplasia. This is a fibroepithelial overgrowth in response to chronic trauma. The cause is an overextended denture flange which transmits the masticatory forces to the soft tissues. This situation often occurs following resorption of the ridges.

The denture hyperplasia may present as one fold or a series of folds like the leaves of a book, which lie in the buccal sulcus either between the alveolus and the denture or along the periphery of the flange.

Treatment. First the irritation is removed by leaving out the denture or easing back the flange. The patient is reviewed after one month and if satisfactory recession has not taken place, it should be excised.

A single hyperplastic fold is removed by grasping it between toothed forceps and cutting through its base. The edges of the wound are then undermined and sutured without altering the depth of the buccal sulcus. Large multi-leaved hyperplasias require excision, and the raw area covered with a split thickness skin graft or a mucosal graft from the cheek or palate. This may be combined with sulcus deepening if necessary.

Cryosurgery has been used and leaves a satisfactory sulcus, but has the disadvantage that no tissue is obtained for biopsy and that the area can be very sore and swollen after operation. An alternative is to excise the hyperplastic tissue using the CO_2 laser. Here the wound is left open and re-epithelialises with minimal contraction or scarring.

Papillary hyperplasia. This presents as multiple small elevations of fibro-epithelial hyperplasia, often associated with chronic candidiasis. Treatment may be with antifungal agents and where indicated surgery. Where the lesion is extensive or there is doubt about its benign nature the area is excised. In less severe cases the small hyperplasias can be removed by crysosurgery or by shaving off the elevations using rotary abrasives.

Increasing the size of the alveolar ridge

Retention and stability depend in part on the orofacial musculature acting on correctly designed dentures, but an important factor is a well formed alveolar ridge which will support adequate vertical flanges on the denture.

The surgical techniques available for increasing the alveolar denture-bearing area are of two kinds: sulcus deepening operations which reposition the soft tissue attachments, particularly of the mandible, and implantation procedures which build up the ridge by introducing under the mucoperio-steum substitutes for the lost alveolar bone.

Sulcus deepening

The size of the denture-bearing area can be increased by deepening the sulci providing there is adequate underlying bone. That this is difficult to do satisfactorily is proved by the number of operations designed to this end, of which only a few are described here. Deepening of the buccal sulcus in the maxilla is seldom necessary as the palate provides a large denture-bearing area. Retention and support for the lower denture would often benefit from deepening of the sulci particularly where muscle attachments have come to lie near the crest of the ridge. Anteriorly the mentalis muscle, laterally the buccinator muscle, and lingually the mylohyoid muscle are involved. To deepen the sulci effectively these muscles must be detached from the mandible and the mucosa made to heal with a new reflection at a lower level. This last is the most difficult part of the operation. It is complicated by the presence of the mental nerve which must be located and preserved from accidental damage.

The procedures available can be considered in four groups.

The mucosa is advanced to line both sides of an extended sulcus (Submucosal vestibuloplasty). An example of this group is Obwegeser's operation. This attempts to divide the muscle attachments and deepen the buccal sulcus without making a flap or leaving raw areas. The procedure is usually performed in the maxilla. Two vertical incisions 1 cm long are made in the buccal sulcus of the canine regions or a single incision in the mid-line. Scissors or a scapel are then passed between mucosa and periosteum. The muscle attachments on the buccal aspect are cut, as far back and upwards as possible, to free the mucosa. This is drawn up and the sulcus maintained by using a denture lined with gutta percha. One or two bone screws in the palate retain the denture for two weeks. Obwegeser's operation has the disadvantage that it is performed blind and if bleeding occurs the new sulcus may be obliterated.

Skin is transplanted to line both sides of an extended sulcus (Buccal inlay). In this operation a pouch is made in the mandibular buccal sulcus which is lined with a split-thickness skin graft from the patient's arm or thigh. An incision is made in the mandibular labial sulcus and a pouch dissected to the required size. This must leave the periosteum intact and attached to bone. An acrylic splint with a gutta percha mould, larger than will eventually be required, is made. Where the skin graft and mucous membrane meet, the mould is grooved so that on healing the ring scar contracts into the groove. The mould is chilled and the skin graft attached to it with the raw surface outwards. This is then placed in the pouch and the splint secured to the mandible with circumferential wires for two weeks.

Skin is transplanted to line one side of an extended sulcus (Lower labial vestibuloplasty). An incision is made along the mandibular alveolar crest from canine to canine. The incision goes through the mucosa but *not* through the mentalis muscle or the periosteum. The mucosal flap is dissected off periosteum and muscles. Care must be taken not to tear the mucosa. Dissection is continued past the reflection, just short of the inner margin of the lip. The mentalis muscle is then divided with a scapel close to the periosteum, which is left undisturbed. The muscle will retract into the deeper tissues. The mucosal flap is repositioned to cover the labial side of the new sulcus and held in position by sutures through the periosteum. A split-thickness skin graft is placed against the raw area of the periosteum with a gutta percha mould on an acrylic splint. In this way, the labial aspect of the new sulcus is lined with mucosa, and the periosteum with the skin graft.

Lowering of floor of mouth and vestibuloplasty. This operation, described by Obwegeser, combines a buccal vestibuloplasty and skin graft with a vestibuloplasty on the lingual aspect of the ridge which heals by secondary epithelialisation. The mucosal flaps on the buccal and lingual sides are held down in the depths of the new sulci by sutures passing under the mandible.

In all vestibuloplasty procedures, the splint or modified denture must be maintained in place for two to three weeks to allow initial healing. During this period, a high standard of oral hygiene is vital. Following removal of the splint, there is a marked tendency for the sulcus to contract. To reduce this, the denture must be modified to extend into the full depth of the sulcus and be worn continuously for several weeks.

Bone substitutes

To increase the height or breadth of the alveolus the chosen material is introduced under the mucoperiosteum to lie directly either on the crest or on the buccal aspect of the alveolus. To avoid an incision line over the graft it is usually introduced into a tunnel made by raising the mucoperiosteum through small vertical incisions in the canine region on each side of the mandible, or a single mid-line incision in the maxilla. The chief difficulty is to obtain sufficient soft tissue cover without producing tension in the mucoperiosteum or reducing the sulcus depth by displacing the mucosal reflection.

A wide variety of materials had been used in the past, many with little success. Biological substances, bone or cartilage, are well tolerated but tend to resorb. Porous ceramic blocks are inert, insoluble and well tolerated but mechanically weak and tend to ulcerate through the mucoperiosteum. Composite materials are easy to fabricate and their properties can be varied to make them resilient and softer to the tissues. However, bone resorption often proceeds beneath them so that the initial gain is later lost. In addition, they often become exposed and infected.

The most reliable bone substitute is calcium hydroxyapatite in the form of small granules of about 1 mm diameter, either solid or porous. This material produced in the laboratory is chemically similar to the inorganic phase of bone. The particles are injected into pockets beneath the periosteum.

Ingrowth of fibrous connective tissue and new bone formation stabilises the mass of particles and produces a firm support for the denture. However there is a tendency for the particles to migrate from the crest of the ridge into the sulcus, with reduction in the height of the augmented ridge and obliteration of the sulcus. To prevent this a tissue-expander inserted into the subperiosteal pocket for two weeks will result in a fibrous tissue-lined tunnel into which the hydroxyapatite particles are injected. This creates a more stable augmentation of the alveolar ridge (Fig. 55, 56).

Fig. 55 Augmentation of resorbed alveolar ridge using hydroxyapatite particles injected, with a special syringe, into a subperiosteal pocket.

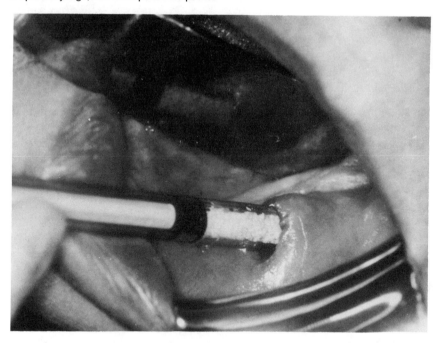

Aids to retention

Aids to retention are only indicated where a specialist prosthetist considers that for psychological or physical reasons the patient is unable to wear either an upper or a lower denture satisfactorily. It is important that the patient clearly understands the procedure and the prognosis.

Implants

In the past, a wide variety of devices were developed to aid denture retention but failed due to infection or bone resorption leading to loosening of the implant. Nowadays more reliable and predictable results can be anticipated from the different varieties available commercially. Careful selection of the implant system is important. They must be constructed of commercially pure titanum. Histological data on the tissue reaction to the implants and the results of follow-up clinical studies should be available.

Endosseous implants are embedded in the jawbone, pass through the mucoperiosteum on the crest of the ridge and may carry single artificial teeth, form a bridge abutment or support a denture. They are usually in two parts. The first inserted into the bone lies flush with the alveolar crest. After a period of three to six months, when bone formation has stabilised the endosseous part, it is exposed and the upper portion screwed into it.

Fig. 56 Top radiograph showing resorbed posterior alveolar ridge. Lower radiograph shows result following augmentation with hydroxyapatite particles.

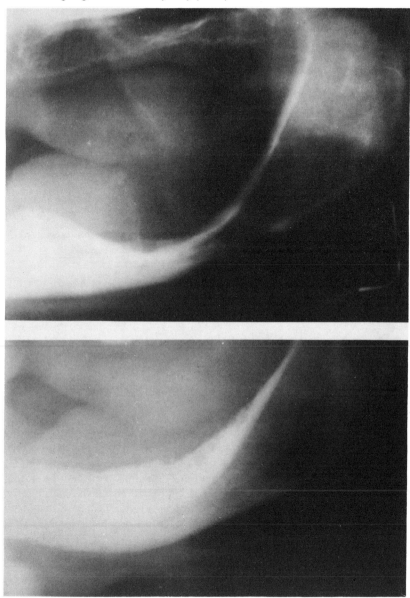

This second part protudes into the mouth to provide retention for the prosthesis. Modern implants are called osseointegrated indicating that they become integrated into the bone. This results in them being firm, stable and able to carry a superstructure onto which a prosthesis may be fitted (Fig. 57).

Fig. 57 Radiographs of osseointegrated titanuim implants with metal bar to retain lower denture.

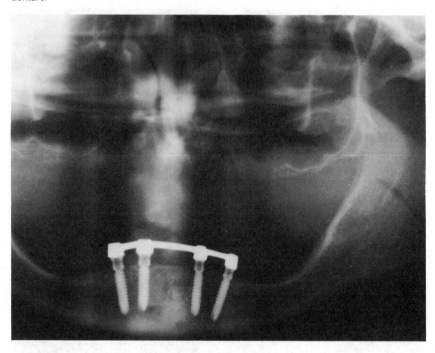

To achieve success careful patient selection, planning and preparation are essential. Patients should be healthy and well motivated, with adequate bone, healthy soft tissues and capable of maintaining a high standard of oral hygiene as plaque and calculus will adhere to implants. The surgical placement of the endosseous part must be carefully carried out and thermal damage to bone avoided when using burs. The mucoperiosteum is initially sutured over the implant and excised after three to six months. The superstructure can then be placed but must not overload the implant.

Osseointegrated implants may be used to replace recently extracted teeth or in long edentulous areas. However, sufficient depth of bone must be present to prevent the implant impinging on adjacent structures such as the nasal floor, maxillary antrum or inferior dental canal. To retain a lower denture, four implants are inserted in the anterior mandible between the mental foramina and are joined together above the mucosa by a gold bar (Fig. 58). Clips inside the denture engage the bar, although the prosthesis is mainly tissue-borne. Alternatively two implants in the lower canine regions may carry retentive anchor attachments which resemble a 'ball-and-socket' system. The patient cleans the exposed part of the implant with a soft toothbrush and toothpaste. Regular follow-up is important to ensure that meticulous oral hygiene is maintained.

Fig. 58 Occlusal view of four titanuim implants in the mandible joined by a metal bar.

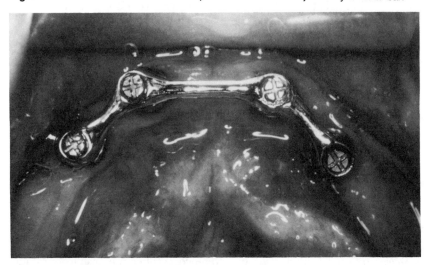

Further reading

Frame, J. W. (1987), 'Hyrdoxyapatite as a biomaterial for alveolar ridge augmentations', *Int. J. O. M. Surg.*, **16**, 642.

Hopkins, R. (1987), *Preprosthetic Oral Surgery*. Wolfe Medical, London.

Howe, G. L. (1985), *Minor Oral Surgery*, 3rd edn. John Wight, Bristol.

XII Treatment of surgical infections about the face

Acute infections in the mouth and face may be caused by traumatic injuries, dental and periodontal disease, dental cysts, or the use of unsterile surgical instruments. Other sources include septic foci in the ear, nose, and throat, on the skin and scalp, and in the salivary glands. The treatment of oral infections requires an understanding of the acute and chronic inflammatory response and how it takes place in the teeth and jaws. For these details textbooks of general and oral pathology should be consulted. The clinical form of the condition will depend on factors which differ for each case.

The causal organism. Dental infections, because the organisms are derived from the flora of the mouth, are often mixed, though staphylococci (especially *Staphylococcus aureus* and *albus*) and streptococci (often responsible for rapidly spreading conditions) are those most commonly isolated. They may also be found in chronic lesions, though the presence of actinomycosis infection should be considered too. Anaerobes may also cause acute or chronic infections in the mouth and care should be taken to culture for these.

Resistance of the patient. This varies from individual to individual and in the same person from time to time. It is related to the well-being of the patient and is lowered in diabetes, metabolic diseases and blood dyscrasias. Where resistance is high and the infection is contained it may resolve, or, if the process does continue, it localises to form pus from the destruction and liquefaction of leucocytes. This is called an abcess. Where the infection cannot be contained spread occurs in the tissue spaces and causes a diffuse, brawny swelling accompanied by systemic upset. This is known as a cellulitis and the rapidity with which it spreads makes it a serious condition demanding energetic treatment.

Local factors. The response to the infection depends on the tissues involved. Bone or tooth pulp react less effectively than does mucous membrane. Where natural drainage can take place quickly the danger of spread is reduced.

Diagnosis

This is made from the history and examination as the five classical signs of acute infection are diagnostic. These are swelling, redness, pain or tenderness, heat, and loss of function. There may be a discharge of pus and the lymphatic nodes draining the area are usually enlarged and tender. Systemic symptoms include a raised temperature, rapid pulse and general malaise.

The typical picture of the acute phase may be altered where antibacterial drugs have been ineffectively used and have not overcome the attack, but have produced a state of balance between the invading bacteria and the patient's defences.

In superficial abscesses, formation of pus causes softening with fluctuation, redness and marked tenderness at the centre of the inflamed area. In deep-seated abscesses of the neck pus may spread widely but fluctuation can be masked by tense, oedematous swelling in the overlying tissues making it difficult to distinguish from a cellulitis. A further rise in an already raised temperature, or a swinging temperature, suggests that suppuration has taken place. The underlying cause (such as a dead tooth) should be sought, though it is not prudent to delay treatment until this has been found.

A careful medical history is taken especially with regard to metabolic or blood diseases. Urine should be tested routinely for sugar. A haemoglobin estimation and differential white cell count should be made in very acute, recurrent, or persistent infections. The erythrocyte sedimentation rate may be estimated.

Radiographs are negative in early acute infections of the jaws unless there has been a previous chronic condition, but after the infection has been present for ten days bone changes may be seen, either as localised periapical areas or as more diffuse changes in osteomyelitis.

Bacteriological investigations are of the utmost importance and no opportunity should be missed to take a specimen for culture.

A bacteriological swab may be used for taking pus either from an extraoral sinus or from an abscess drained through an extraoral incision, providing that the skin and surrounding area has been thoroughly cleansed beforehand. However swabs taken inside the mouth appear to be very liable to contamination from the saliva so that growths obtained are often reported as 'mixed oral flora'. Where collections of pus have not been opened to the mouth it is better to take a specimen for culture by aspiration. The mucosa is first thoroughly cleaned and dried and an aspirating syringe used to draw off a small quantity of pus for culture. This should be immediately sealed from drying and contamination from the air. It should be labelled with the patient's name, number and the date. It is sent, accompanied by details of the history and any antibiotic therapy, to a hospital bacteriologist. He will culture the organisms, identify them and give an indication of drugs to which the bacteria will be sensitive.

Principles of treatment of acute infections

General measures

The general care of patients has been discussed in Chapter II.

Rest. Rest in bed is advisable where the temperature is raised. When there is gross swelling of the neck, or the patient is toxic, he should be admitted to hospital.

Fluids. These are given copiously to combat dehydration, a complication of high fever. Circulating toxins are diluted and their excretion encouraged by a big turnover of water.

Diet. This should consist of easily digested proteins and carbohydrates (Chaper II).

Control of infection. Antibacterial drugs are not always necessary in the treatment of infections. Drainage and applications of heat may be enough to enable the patient to overcome the condition and antibiotics must not be prescribed to replace or delay these local measures. Where the infection is spreading or there are signs of systematic involvement such as general malaise, a flushed dry skin or a raised body temperature the immediate use of antibiotics is indicated. Unfortunately it is often impossible at this stage to take a culture or, where this can be done, to wait for results. Antibiotics must then be prescribed blind. The drug of choice is pencillin because it is in general use and known to be effective in dental infections. Where the patient is hypersensitive to penicillin, erythromycin may be used. Should anaerobic bacteria be the suspected cause, metronidazole should be considered.

Antibiotics must be prescribed for a minimum course of three days in big doses which quickly obtain a high blood level and then maintain it. With penicillin this is best achieved with an initial loading dose of 600 mg benzyl penicillin and 600 mg procaine penicillin at twelve-hourly intervals. Oral penicillin may be less satisfactory but can be given in doses of 500 mg at six-hourly intervals. Erythromycin is started with a dose of 500 mg followed by 250 mg six-hourly, by mouth. Unless positive bacteriological evidence is obtained that the organism is resistant, no change should be made in the course of antibiotics for forty-eight hours to give it time to be effective. After that if there is no improvement a change may be made for one with which organisms do not generally have cross resistance.

Local measures

Oral hygiene. A high standard of oral hygiene must be maintained.

Increase in blood supply to the part. In the mouth and on the face this is stimulated by heat. When applied intraorally as hot salt water mouth baths this penetrates only 1 mm into the tissues and is rapidly removed by the circulation. However, the local vasodilatation produced does hasten the inflammatory response and, as a result , the infection localises and points. Heat is contraindicated in bone infections before drainage has taken place, particularly in the mandible where it may cause an osteomyelitis.

Drainage. Localisation of pus (pointing) is indicated by reddening of the skin, fluctuation and a point of maximum tenderness. When this occurs the pus must be let out and a surgical incision leaves much less scarring than if pus bursts through the skin spontaneously. Drainage, to be effective, must be provided at the lowest point of the abscess. A drain (Fig. 15) should always be inserted to keep the opening patent for as long as the discharge continues. In cellulitis drainage is not established until the condition has localised, usually after three or four days, but where a brawny, spreading swelling of the floor of the mouth and neck might involve the larynx and jeopardise the airway, surgery, which will reduce the tension in the tissue spaces, should not be withheld.

Incisions in the mucous membrane are made about 3 cm long and parallel to the occlusal surface of the teeth. Smaller incisions are ineffective. Where satisfactory dependent drainage can only be obtained through the skin, this should be incised extraorally, carefully avoiding the branches of the facial nerve. Where the abscess is deep and a free discharge is not obtained by simple incision through the skin, Hilton's method is used. In this a pair of fine sinus forceps are inserted closed into the wound and opened slowly but firmly to separate the soft tissue planes. The forceps are then withdrawn *open* to avoid damaging nerves or vessels by closing them blind. This procedure is repeated till the abscess is reached and pus discharges. In dental infections an area of rough cortical bone can be felt on the mandible or maxilla where the periosteum has been raised.

Rest of the inflamed part.   This important principle in treating acute infections is not easily applied to the mouth. Trismus does, however, produce enforced rest.

Removal of the cause.   The need to remove the underlying cause is obvious but when to remove it, more difficult. In well-localised minor infections it can be done immediately and may cure the condition. In other cases it may be contraindicated as a first measure owing to the danger of spreading infection.

Timing.   The decision when to do various procedures is of great importance and requires considerable experience. Where there is an acute infection with a high temperature, treatment should be started immediately with antibacterial drugs, but if pus has localised this must be drained without delay and sensitivity tests made which will take at least forty-eight hours to give results. Therefore, antibacterial drugs are best started blind, before drainage is instituted, and continued until the results of the sensitivity tests are available. In conditions where trismus may develop and make anaesthesia hazardous, incision and drainage should not be delayed. In trismus the mouth must on no account be racked open with a gag lest infection be spread through the tissue spaces. As soon as the acute phase has passed the cause should be removed.

Maintainance of airway.   Infections in the neck may cause oedema of the glottis with acute respiratory embarrassment which must be relieved by performing a tracheostomy. In all acute swellings where swallowing is difficult patients should be watched for signs of difficulty in breathing and everything necessary for an emergency tracheostomy should be at hand. Where there is *any respiratory difficulty no attempt should be made to give a general anaesthetic* lest respiratory arrest occur when the accessory muscles of respiration stop functioning. Anaesthesia may be induced after tracheostomy.

Pericoronitis

This is inflammation about the crown of an erupting or partly erupted, but impacted, tooth. Though rare in the maxilla, it is common in the mandible and is particularly associated with the lower third molar.

This tooth often has a chronic pericoronitis from the time its crown communicates with the mouth. Sooner or later an acute attack supervenes, often precipitated by the upper third molar biting the lower gum flap (Fig. 59). The patient complains of pain and tenderness in the gum flap and a nasty taste from discharging pus. When severe there is swelling of the floor of mouth and face, with trismus. There may be difficulty in swallowing and a raised temperature.

Diagnosis. This is made after confirming the presence of the unerupted tooth with radiographs, and eliminating apical or periodontal disease in neighbouring teeth.

Treatment. This is in two stages, directed first to the infection and second to the unerupted tooth.

For the acute inflammation, hourly hot salt water mouth baths to be held over the affected gum are ordered. Where the temperature is raised or trismus is present antibacterial drugs are prescribed. In pericoronitis of the lower third molar it is essential to eliminate trauma from the upper third molar. Where the upper tooth is non-functional it can be extracted at once under local anaesthesia, providing access is satisfactory. Where the tooth is functional the cusps may be ground clear of the gum flap or a temporary bite-raising applicance provided. With this care the infection should resolve but can be complicated by an abscess or cellulitis, the treatment of which is described below.

Fig. 59 As it is often difficult to see if the upper third molar is biting on the inflamed gingival flap over a partly erupted lower third molar, a dental probe may be placed distal to the upper third molar and drawn forward over its occlusal surface with the teeth in occlusion. This will not be possible where the upper cusps are in contact with the swollen gum flap.

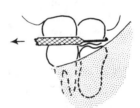

The surgical treatment of the unerupted tooth is best delayed until the acute phase, particularly the trismus, has resolved, which may take some two to three weeks. Consideration should be given to the use of an antibiotic cover for the extraction and the socket is packed open. Excision of the gum flap for pericoronitis has been practised but the results are unsatisfactory and it is to be condemned except where the tooth will erupt into occlusion.

Acute periapical abscess without soft tissue involvement

Periapical infection from dead teeth or periodontal disease may either be contained, and present as a low-grade chronic condition or apical granuloma with mild symptoms, or may suppurate to form an acute periapical abscess.

Diagnosis. The patient with an acute periapical abscess complains of severe pain and the affected tooth feels raised in its socket. At first the pain may be eased by biting on the tooth but later it becomes exquisitely tender to touch. Examination at an early stage shows no involvement of the oral mucosa or soft tissue and systemic symptoms are usually absent.

Treatment. Where it is hoped to retain the tooth, the root canal is opened through the crown to provide drainage and access for root canal therapy. Otherwise the tooth may be extracted under a general anaesthetic, or antibiotics given to reduce the infection. Local anaesthesia can then be used for the extraction, but should be avoided in the acute condition as it may be ineffective, and infiltration anaesthesia is certainly contraindicated lest it cause a spread of infection.

Subperiosteal abscess and spread into soft tissues

Pus from the acute periapical abscess will take the line of least resistance through the medullary bone to point on the nearest epithelial surface. This is usually the buccal aspect on either the maxilla or mandible as the alveolar bone is thinner on this side. The pus may break through the bone either above or below the attachment of the buccinator muscle and this determines whether it discharges into the mouth or through the soft tissues on to the skin of the face (Fig. 60).

Certain roots are placed nearer the lingual or palatal cortical plates and pus may go that way. In the maxilla the lateral incisor and the palatal roots of the molar teeth give rise to palatal abscesses. In the mandible, if pus tracks lingually, it is the relationship of the roots to the attachment of the mylohyoid muscle that determines where it will discharge. Thus the apices of the lower third molar, and sometimes the second molar, lie below (superficial to) the insertion of mylohyoid and their apical abscesses tend to point through the skin. The rest of the mandibular root apices lie above (deep to) the mylohyoid and pus from them leaves the bone above this muscle to escape the floor of the mouth.

Fig. 60 Spread of infection: (a) Coronal section through the tissue spaces of the face and neck. Note A the maxillary sinus, B the buccinator muscle, M the mylohyoid muscle, S the submandibular salivary gland. Spaces shown are (1) the submandibular and (2) the sublingual. (b) Transverse section through the tissue spaces of the face and neck. Note A the parotid salivary gland, B the buccinator muscle, C the superior constrictor muscle, M the masseter muscle, P the medial pterygoid muscle and (1) the carotid sheath. Spaces shown are (2) the lateral pharnygeal, (3) the retro-pharyngeal, (4) the submasseteric, (5) the pterygomandibular.

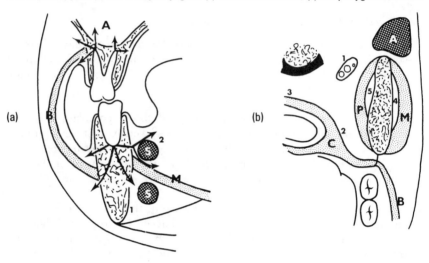

Periapical abscesses can discharge through the root canal or the periodontal membrane, and, in the maxilla, from anterior teeth into the floor of the nose, or from molars and second premolars into the maxillary sinus (Fig. 60).

Diagnosis. All the cardinal signs of acute inflammation are present, often with mild systemic symptoms. First a tense, very painful subperiosteal swelling is seen near the tooth with some oedema of the face. The acute pain improves when pus is released through the mucoperiosteum into the mouth or through the periosteum into the soft tissues of the face and neck.

Treatment. When the abscess is accompanied by facial swelling which is neither hard and brawny, as in a cellulitis, nor fluctuant like pus but is obviously an inflammatory oedema, the treatment is as described for an acute periapical abscess. Pus, if present under the mucoperiosteum, will not drain back through bone after the extraction and the abscess must be incised and drained. Wherever systemic symptoms are present these procedures are better completed under an antibacterial cover.

Infections of the face and neck

Spread of infection in the soft tissues of the face takes place through the lymphatic system or along the fascial and muscular planes.

Lymphatic drainage. The lymphatic system is an important part of the body's defence against infection, but is itself involved in the condition. The lymphatic vessels draining the scalp and the skin of the face pass into the superficial groups of nodes arranged in a circle round the head. These are the occipital, posterior auricular, parotid, and facial nodes. Efferent vessels from these pass down to the superior glands of the deep cervical chain.

The lower, lip, the incisor region of the mandible, and the anterior part of the tongue and floor of the mouth drain into the submental lymph nodes, which lie between the anterior bellies of the two digastric muscles. Lymph passes from them into the submandibular nodes or direct to the deep cervical chain. The remaining lymphatic vessels of the lips, cheeks, tongue and jaws drain directly into the submandibular lymph nodes, which lie in the submandibular triangle, and thence into the deep cervical nodes which accompany the internal jugular vein in the neck. Lymph from the anterior part of the mouth passes into the lower group of nodes in this chain, and that from the posterior part into the upper group. A large node of the superior group (the jugulodigastric), situated at the level of the posterior belly of the digastric muscle, is one of the first to become enlarged and palpable in pathological conditions of the mouth and tonsil.

The lymphatics and lymph nodes show a response which varies with the severity of the infection. In acute infection the lymphatic channels may become inflamed (lymphangitis). More commonly the organisms and their toxins reach the lymph node which becomes enlarged and tender (lymphadenitis). In virulent infections suppuration and abscess formation may occur in the node. Enlarged lymph nodes from causes other than dental infection must be considered; the differential diagnosis of these will be found in medical textbooks.

Spread through the muscular and fascial planes. Spread of infection takes place through the potential spaces, normally filled with loose areolar tissue, which lie between muscles, bones and viscera. These are covered by condensations of fascia which form strong fibrous sheets, the most important of which is the deep cervical fascia.

The deep cervical fascia. The superficial layer encloses the neck and prevents deep infections pointing easily on to the skin.

It arises below from the scapula, the clavicle and the manubrium sterni, and sweeps up the neck as a continuous tube attached posteriorly to ligamentum nuchae and anteriorly to the hyoid bone. At the lower border of the mandible it divides to be attached lingually to the mylohyoid line and buccally to the outer aspect of the mandible. The space so formed is the submandibular space in which the lower part of the submandibular salivary gland is sited (Fig. 60a). From the buccal aspect of the mandible the fascia is reflected up on to the zygomatic arch and posteriorly ensheaths the parotid gland, is inserted into the mastoid process and the superior nuchal line on the skull. It forms invaginations into the neck, *the pretracheal fascia*, a continuation from the deep surface, which invests the trachea and thyroid gland, *the prevertebral fascia* which lies anterior to the prevertebral muscles, and the *carotid sheath* round the great vessels of the neck. All these extend down into the thorax and can provide a pathway for spread of infection into the mediastinum.

Sublingual spaces. On the medial aspect of the mandible above (deep to) the mylohyoid there are two sublingual spaces. The more superficial lies between the mylohyoid and geniohyoid muscles, the deeper between geniohyoid and genioglossus. Both spaces are continuous across the midline and are bounded by the insertion of these muscles into the hyoid bone. Infection can track laterally across the floor of the mouth, or back to cause an inflammatory oedema of the larynx with respiratory embarrassment. The upper (deep) part of the submandibular salivary gland lies in the sublingual space and the gland curves round the posterior edge of the mylohyoid muscle into the submandibular space, thus providing a connection between submandibular and sublingual spaces (Fig. 60a).

The pterygomandibular space. This is the space between the medical aspect of the ascending ramus of the mandible and the medical pterygoid muscle and is limited above by the lateral pterygoid muscle. It communicates with the lateral pharyngeal and the infratemporal spaces (Fig. 60b).

The lateral pharyngeal space. The boundaries of this space are medially the superior constrictor of the pharynx, laterally the medial pterygoid muscle and anteriorly the pterygomandibular raphe where the fascia covering the superior constrictor is reflected on to the medial pterygoid muscle. Posteriorly it is bounded by the styloid process and the stylohyoid and stylopharyngeus muscles along which infection may pass down to the larynx. It is also in close relation to the carotid sheath. The space communicates with both sublingual and submandibular spaces round the submandibular salivary gland, the posterior part of which protrudes into the lateral pharyngeal space.

The submandibular gland therefore plays an important part in the spread of infection as it links the submandibular, the sublingual, and lateral pharyngeal spaces (Fig. 60).

The retropharyngeal space. This lies between the constrictors of the pharynx and the prevertebral muscles. It therefore connects the right and left lateral pharygeal spaces posteriorly (Fig. 60b).

The infratemporal space. It is bounded anteriorly by the tuberosity of the maxilla, medially by the lateral pterygoid plate and the inferior belly of the lateral pterygoid muscle, and laterally by the tendon of temporalis muscle and the coronoid process.

The submasseteric space. This is a potential space between the masseter muscle and the outer plate of the mandible.

Maxillary infections

Where pus points buccally above the buccinator it will form an abscess in the cheek and may spread over a wide area as there is nothing to contain it. Those from the anterior teeth cause an infraorbital abscess which is serious because thrombosis of the facial vein may follow. This vessel has anastomosis with orbital veins which drain into the cavernous sinus. In this way infection may pass from the face into the cavernous sinus.

Abscesses in the cheek may point anywhere on the face and when drained the incision is made parallel to the branches of the facial nerve. Infection of the infratemporal space may be caused by posterior superior dental nerve injections given behind the tuberosity of the maxilla or by spread from the maxillary third molar tooth. This space may be drained intraorally through the buccal sulcus lateral and posterior to the tuberosity.

Mandibular infections

Spread of infection buccally, below the attachment of the buccinator, causes a swelling in the cheek over the lateral aspect of the mandible, but the inferior border of the bone remains palpable if the submandibular space is not involved. Incision for drainage may have to be made over the lateral aspect of the mandible.

An infection in the submandibular space gives rise to swelling over the lower border of the mandible and into the neck. It is drained by an incision parallel with the lower border of the mandible and about 2 cm below it to avoid the mandibular branch of the facial nerve and the facial vessels.

The sublingual spaces are involved when spread takes place above the mylohyoid into the floor of the mouth which becomes swollen and raised with difficulty in swallowing. These may be drained by an incision in the floor of the mouth but, if the submandibular space is also involved, an extraoral approach is more satisfactory.

Infection of the pterygomandibular space, with symptoms of trismus and pain on swallowing, may follow an inferior dental nerve injection or spread of infection from the lower third molar tooth. This space and the submandibular space communicate with the lateral pharyngeal space which, if involved, gives rise to swelling in the lateral wall of the oropharynx, and mesial and posterior to the angle of the mandible accompanied by trismus and difficulty in swallowing.

The lateral pharyngeal, and through it the pterygomandibular space, may be drained by an incision made 2 cm below the angle of the mandible. In those rare cases where only the pterygomandibular space is affected it may be opened by incising down the anterior border of the ascending ramus intraorally.

Infection from the lower third molar teeth may also occasionally track buccally either under the skin superficial to masseter or less often into the submassetric space (Fig. 60b).

Ludwig's angina. This term is loosely used to indicate a cellulitis of the submandibular and sublingual spaces on both sides which may also spread back to the lateral pharyngeal spaces and down to the larynx to cause oedema of the glottis and asphyxia. Characteristically the tongue is lifted up and forward by the swelling to protrude between the teeth through such opening as is possible (Fig. 61). Trismus may be severe and the swelling is 'board' hard. There is danger of spread to the thorax by the carotid sheath and so to the cavernous sinus by the pterygoid venous plexus. In severe cases a tracheostomy may be required.

The cellulitis is treated with antibiotics and external incisions with through-and through drains into the floor of the mouth. Incisions are made bilaterally at the lower border of the mandible in the first or second molar region and the tissue planes dissected by Hilton's method until the floor of the mouth is reached, when a second incision is made. Corrugated rubber drains are then drawn through and sutured into place with one end protruding on the skin and the other in the mouth. Pus is seldom found but the congestion may be relieved.

Osteomyelitis

Osteomyelitis is an infection involving all the layers of the bone in which widespread necrosis may occur. In the adult the maxillary complex is seldom affected as the thin plates of bone have a rich blood supply, but it

Fig. 61 Patient with Ludwig's angina. Note the tongue protruding between the teeth and the inflammatory response over the upper part of the thorax.

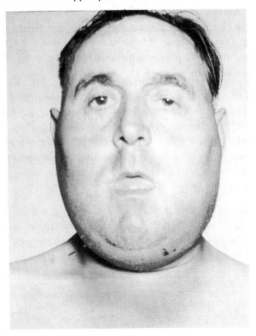

is occasionally seen in the anterior part of the palate where the bone is thicker. Osteomyelitis of the mandible is more common and is usually dental or traumatic in origin, though it may arise as a blood-borne infection.

The factors which favour its development are highly virulent organisms, low resistance of the patient and lack of drainage. The latter is important clinically as it can be rectified by surgery. In osteomyelitis the pus, instead of passing through the bone along a narrow track to point in the soft tissue, spreads through the medulla and reaches the cortical plate at several points to lift the periosteum from the bone and deprive sometimes large areas of their blood supply. Eventually the pus discharges through a sinus, and if drainage is satisfactory the condition enters a chronic stage. In an attempt to limit the infection dead bone is separated by osteoclasts and walled off by granulation tissue. Repair and support of the weakened bone is started by the osteoblasts of the periosteum which lay down a new layer of bone, the involucrum. This is seldom very marked in the jaws, although it does occur. Discharge continues until the sequestra are removed. Wherever drainage is inadequate slow spread may continue indefinitely with the formation of new sequestra.

Diagnosis. The symptoms of acute osteomyelitis are those of an acute infection with severe pain and a raised temperature. Teeth in the affected area are tender to percussion and become loose. In the mandible there is loss of sensation in the mental nerve which is often intermittent. Swelling of the face, if not present initially, soon follows. Eventually pus discharges and sinuses are formed, at the bottom of which bare, rough bone may be felt.

Today, antibiotic therapy has reduced the incidence of acute osteomyelitis. More commonly patients present with chronic inflammatory swellings complicated by subacute episodes which settle with a course of antibacterial drugs. Where these are prescribed for too short a period the symptoms may be suppressed without the disease being cured. The destruction of bone may be extensive if this situation has continued for some period of time.

Radiographs are at first negative unless there has been a long-standing chronic infection. Normally changes are seen only ten days after the start of the disease and present as irregular radiolucent areas (Fig. 62). Sequestra later show as radiopaque bodies surrounded by a radiolucent zone. Destruction may predipose to a pathological fracture which can be seen on radiographs.

Treatment. Patients with acute osteomyelitis should be admitted to hospital immediately, and treatment directed to controlling the infection with high doses of antibiotics, and to establishing drainage through an external incision. The drilling of holes into the bone is neither necessary nor advisable, nor should any but very loose and dead teeth be extracted. The use of heat is contraindicated lest it lead to further spread in the bone. This treatment alone may cause the acute phase to resolve and even loose teeth may tighten and be found to have remained vital. Antibiotic therapy should be continued for a fortnight after the disease has apparently settled, which may take several weeks.

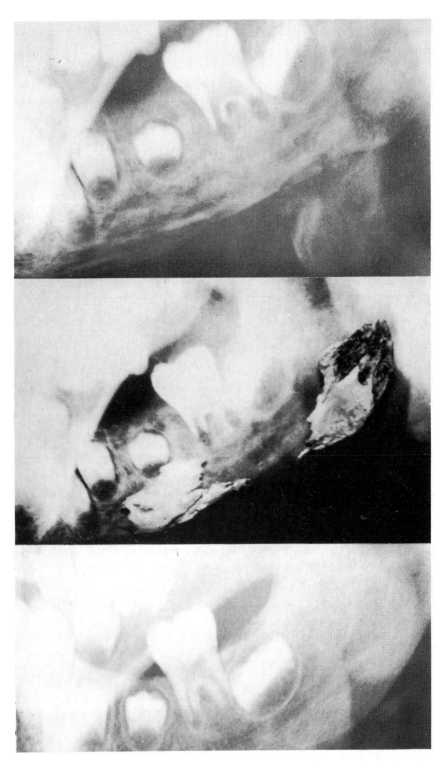

Sequestrectomy. Treatment in the chronic phase consists of administering antibiotics, maintaining drainage, and sequestrectomy, which should always be done under an antibacterial cover. For satisfactory removal sequestra should be lying loose, which on radiographs is suggested by a clear radiolucent line round the dead bone. Otherwise at operation it is difficult to judge the line of separation and dead bone may be left or healthy tissue needlessly traumatised. A splint is prepared before operation and, if destruction is extensive, put in place to support the mandible. Sequestra lying above the inferior dental canal may be removed through an intraoral transalveolar approach, and the wound packed open. Those below the canal are taken out through an extraoral incision below the lower border of the mandible. When a sinus opens on the skin of the neck this should be incorporated in the incision, and a seeker inserted in the sinus to assist in localising the sequestrum. The flap raised, cortical bone is removed sufficiently to lift out the dead bone, and exuberant septic granulations are gently curetted to expose healthy bleeding bone. Drains are put in place.

Mowlem's decorticetomy. The thick cortical plate over the lower border and buccal aspect of the mandible has a poor blood supply and is very vulnerable to infection. Mowlem's operation removes this bone from over the diseased area, allows granulations to grow in and speeds recovery.

Splints are prepared and fitted, and an antibacterial cover prescribed. At operation an incision is made over the affected area 2.5 cm below the lower border of the mandible. The facial vessels are ligated where necessary. The lower border of the mandible is exposed and with burs (chisels may fracture the bone) the lower and outer cortical plates are removed (Fig. 62). Sequestra and granulations are curetted out to leave healthy bleeding bone. The lingual plate is left intact. The area is saucerised, drains are inserted (tube drains are used to irrigate the wound) and the wound closed. Splints are left in place for a month to allow new bone to form and support the mandible. Antibacterial drugs are continued for a fortnight post-operatively. This operation dramatically cuts short the course of the disease and reduces the destruction that may occur from slow spread during the chronic phase.

Acute maxillary infection in infants

This is a rare, acute, staphylococcal infection which affects infants a few weeks old. It occurs usually in the maxilla and the possible causes are birth trauma, mouth abrasions or blood-borne infection.

Diagnosis. The disease, which is of rapid onset, has all the signs of an acute infection, the child being very ill with a high temperature. The cheek is

---

Fig. 62 (*Opposite page*) Osteomyelitis in a child. *Top:* lateral oblique radiograph of mandible to show osteomyelitis. *Middle:* part of the bone removed by decorticectomy superimposed on the lateral oblique radiograph. *Bottom:* six months later, showing normal state of bone with unerupted teeth which later erupted satisfactorily.

swollen, and the eye closed, pus may discharge from intraoral sinuses over the maxilla or down the nose. The partly calcified teeth of the maxilla are cut off from the blood supply and become sequestra. Occasionally the thicker bony margins of the maxilla (infraorbital margin) may also sequestrate. Radiographs are valueless, as the maxilla at this state is virtually just a 'bag of teeth' with only thin bony plates.

Treatment. The patient is admitted to hospital and should be placed under the care of a paediatrician for the supervision of his general day-to-day care. Treatment of the acute infection is with antibiotics and drainage. Many settle with this treatment alone if caught early. Sequestrated teeth maintain a chronic discharge later and require extraction.

Acute osteomyelitis in children

Acute osteomyelitis, chiefly of the mandible, may occur in young children following exanthematous fevers, tonsillitis, sinusitis or middle ear disease. The symptoms and course of the disease are the same as in adult osteomyelitis and unerupted teeth are frequently exfoliated. The situation is more urgent, however, as spread to the growth centres and into the condyle can cause severe deformity in the mandible and ankylosis of the joint.

Treatment. This follows the same pattern as for adult osteomyelitis.

Chronic infections about the jaws

Chronic periapical abscess

An acute periapical abscess can become chronic if the cause is not removed and it drains through a sinus. It may be subject to acute exacerbations whenever the sinus is blocked. Treatment is by extraction or root filling and apicectomy. Chronic sinuses on the skin are excised to avoid ugly residual scars.

Tuberculous infection of the jaws

Infections of the mouth by *Mycobacterium tuberculosis* are almost invariably secondary to tuberculosis elsewhere, usually the lungs. The mouth may become infected from sputum or by haematogenous spread. Cervical tuberculous adenitis occurs without infection at other sites and should be considered in the differential diagnosis of enlarged non-painful lymph nodes.

Diagnosis. Tuberculous ulcers in the mouth are diagnosed by culturing smears for Mycobacterium tuberculosis, and the chest should be radiographed for other foci. Osteomyelitis can occur and is characterised by a long-standing localised swelling which is tender and may soften to discharge on the skin at the lower border of the mandible. Sequestra are formed and secondary infection may occur.

Treatment. This is first directed to the general care of the patient. The local condition is treated by antibacterials, drainage and sequestrectomy where necessary.

Syphilis of the jaws

Lesions occur in the tertiary stage in two forms, gumma which occurs chiefly in the maxilla, and a diffuse osteitis in the mandible. Gumma in the palate usually starts in the submucosa or periosteum, spreading to and destroying the bone of the hard palate, in the midline. This can be demonstrated radiographically. The resulting ulceration may resemble carcinoma and should be differentially diagnosed from it with the use of serology and biopsy. In the mandible the more diffuse form may mimic acute osteomyelitis without malaise and raised temperature.

Treatment. This is directed towards the underlying disease and surgical intervention is contraindicated owing to the danger of secondary infection and osteomyelitis. If the medical history reveals evidence of previous syphilis, extraction should be carried out under antibiotic cover to avoid the occurrence of syphylitic osteomyelitis.

Actinomycosis

This is a chronic infection caused by *Actinomyces israelii* which may affect the face and neck, the lungs or abdomen.

Diagnosis. The patient complains of a 'board' hard, lumpy swelling usually over the angle of the mandible. It is sometimes bluish in colour and tends to form multiple sinuses which discharge pus containing 'sulphur granules'. These, if examined microscopically, show the organisms.

Sometimes the disease occurs as a mixed infection and presents as a typical acute abscess which fails to clear up normally. In these cases frequent anaerobic cultures should be made as there is often difficulty in isolating the organism and the diagnosis cannot be definitely established without a positive culture. Rarely is the bone also involved.

Treatment. Antibacterial drugs are prescribed, for a period of four to six weeks. Surgery is limited to draining superficial lesions, but if bone is involved the affected area may be curetted, packed open and the teeth involved extracted.

Further reading

Birn, H. (1972), 'Spread of dental infections', *Dent. Practit.*, **22**, 347.
Melville, T. H. and Russell, C. (1975), *Microbiology for Dental Students.* Heinemann, London.
Mowlem, R. (1945), 'Osteomyelitis of the jaw', *Proc. Roy. Soc. Med.*, **38**, 452.
Seward, G. R., Harris, M. and McGowan, D. A. (1987), *Killey and Kay's Outline of Oral Surgery*, 2nd edn. John Wright, Bristol.

XIII Treatment of cysts of the mouth

Dental or periodontal cysts. These form from the epithelial cells or rests of Malassez which are the remnants of Hertwig's sheath. They remain throughout life, scattered in clusters, in the periodontal membrane. Chronic infection may stimulate them to proliferate and form epithelial lined cysts in the jaws. These occur chiefly over the apex of a dead tooth, but may occasionally be found on its lateral aspect, when they are called lateral periodontal cysts.

Residual cysts. These occur in edentulous areas of the jaws and are dental cysts believed to have been present before the dead tooth was extracted and which continue to grow.

Dentigerous cysts. These form between the reduced enamel epithelium of the follicle around a developing tooth and its crown.

Eruption cysts. These are cysts forming over erupting teeth. Those over deciduous or permanent teeth with no deciduous predecessor are believed to originate from the cells of the enamel organ. Where there has been a deciduous predecessor the epithelial rests of Malassez from this tooth could give rise to one of these cysts.

The above cysts of dental origin are believed to increase in size either from continual liquefaction of their shed cells (which forms the cholesterol that gives the contents a characteristic golden appearance) or as a result of the positive osmotic pressure of the hypertonic contents which draws water in from the tissues.

Keratocysts (primordial cysts). These are said to arise from the dental lamina or from the enamel organ of a tooth germ. Their lining is of well-differentiated epithelium which may show ortho- or para-keratosis. They are believed to increase in size by mural division. Beneath the epithelium is thin fibrous tissue which is easily torn and satellite cysts lying outside the main body of the lesion are often found. For these reasons keratocysts are well known to be difficult to eradicate and likely to recur after treatment. The recurrence rate has been reported to be 20–60 per cent. The complete removal of all the lining of these cysts to avoid recurrence is of great importance. Their contents have less soluble protein (less than 5 g per 100 ml) than dental cysts.

Diagnosis

History

The patient often gives no history, as many of the smaller dental cysts are discovered only when dead or heavily filled teeth are radiographed. Larger cysts may cause swelling of the jaw or face which in the edentulous may be associated with difficulty in wearing dentures. In the mandible, pressure on the inferior dental nerve almost never gives rise to mental anaesthesia or paraesthesia, an important point is differentiation from tumours. Occasionally cysts reach such proportions that excessive resorption of bone leads to pathological fracture. Eventually the majority of cysts become infected with acute symptoms and, in those which have expanded into the soft tissues, an increase in the swelling.

Examination

An eruption cyst presents as a small blue swelling in the gum over an unerupted tooth. Uninfected dental, residual, or dentigerous cysts are painless and non-tender on palpation. When they are small and enclosed in bone they show no change in the form of the alveolus. Larger cysts cause a marked, smooth, rounded expansion of the bone, which may be reduced to a thin layer of cortical plate. This, if pressed, is resilient and may give rise to egg-shell crackling. In the mandible this expansion is said to take place buccally only, but occasionally it is seen lingually as well. Where the cyst has invaded the soft tissues the swelling is found to be fluctuant and a definite thrill can be made to pass through it. At this stage, if the mucous membrane covering is thin, it will have a bluish colour. Infected cysts have all the classical signs of acute infection and may present with a sinus discharging pus.

Missing teeth must be charted and the standing teeth carefully examined for caries, periodontal disease and mobility. A dentigerous cyst may be suspected where a tooth is missing from the arch without any history of previous extraction. Dead and root-filled teeth are associated with dental cysts. The vitality of all teeth near the lesion must be tested with an electric pulp tester and the results compared with similar teeth on the unaffected side. If there is any delay between diagnosis and operation these tests should be repeated immediately before operation, for cysts not only arise from dead teeth but their expansion may also devitalise adjacent teeth.

Keratocysts may present like dental cysts but occur most commonly in the lower third molar region or distal to it and invade the ascending ramus extensively. They tend to expand anteroposteriorly in the medullary bone of the mandible and reach some size with minimal expansion of the cortical plate. Diagnosis may result from an infective episode or as a result of discovery on a scanning radiograph (Fig. 63).

Radiography

Intraoral apical films usually suffice for small cysts. Larger ones may need extraoral and occlusal views of the jaws to show their full extent. This is demonstrated by radiographs taken in two planes, as treatment planning depends on a clear understanding of their size and their relationship to those vital structures on which they may encroach.

Cysts appear as rounded, radiolucent areas sharply demarcated from normal bone by a thin, radiopaque, limiting line of compact bone (Fig. 63). This

Fig. 63 *Above left:* lateral oblique radiograph showing a keratocyst of the left mandible. *Above right:* follow-up film of same patient one year after surgery to show new bone formation. *Below:* Orthopantomograph of marsupialised cyst with pack in situ.

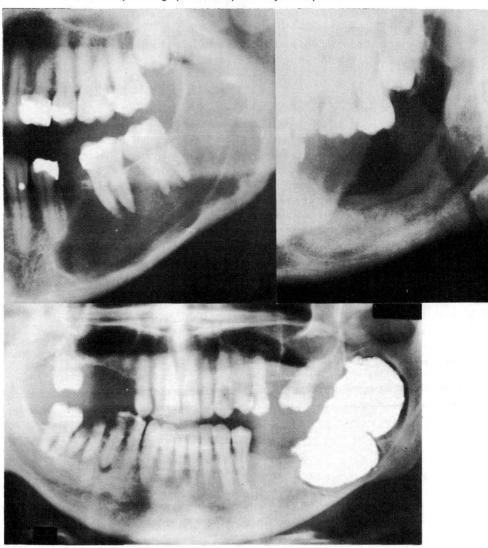

line is not usually present on radiographs of apical granulomas and is often absent or hazy round infected cysts. Apical periodontal cysts are associated with the roots of dead teeth and may throw a shadow over, or displace, the roots of neighbouring teeth which, though apparently involved, may yet still be vital. Dental cysts, particularly the keratocyst, if loculated may simulate ameloblastoma or central giant cell reparative granuloma.

In the maxilla it is sometimes difficult to tell whether a radiolucent area is a cyst or a locule of the maxillary sinus. Therefore it is necessary to compare the radiographs with those of the opposite side; if a similar locule is present the radiolucent area is probably part of the sinus. If all the teeth are standing and vital, a cyst is unlikely to be present, Finally, where doubts still exist, the area may be aspirated and if air, not fluid, is withdrawn it is certainly part of the maxillary sinus.

Radiopaque fluids. Where the size and relations of a cyst are in doubt its contents may be aspirated and radiopaque fluid introduced. In large cavities it may only be possible to replace a proportion of the cyst contents, but the boundaries can be defined by taking radiographs with the head tilted in different positions so that the radiopaque medium lies against the doubtful margins.

Aspiration

An aspirating syringe with a broad bore needle is used, as the contents can be quite thick. Uninfected cysts should not be aspirated more than twenty-four hours before operation to avoid introducing infection.In those covered by thick bone it may be better delayed till, at operation, a flap has been laid back and bone removed.

All cysts of any size should be aspirated before operation. It is an important diagnostic measure which can save the surgeon much embarrassment from accidentally opening a solid tumour, or worse a central haemangioma. Microscopic examination of the aspirate may show the presence of cholesterol.

Further only in this way may a keratocyst be differentiated from other odontogenic cysts before operation. This is done by electrophoresis of the aspirate which for keratocysts will show less than 5 g in 100 ml of soluble protein whereas other dental cysts will have quantities similar to that in the patient's serum.

Differential diagnosis

Many lesions may resemble cysts. These include solitary bone cyst, aneurysmal bone cyst, central giant cell granuloma, ameloblastoma, and certain general diseases such as osteitis fibrosa cystica. Where doubt exists, blood chemistry, aspiration and biopsy should be performed.

Assessment

This includes an estimation of their size and, particularly in the mandible, the extent of bone resorption. Should there be a risk of a pathological fracture, suitable splints must be prepared. Many cysts, however, which on lateral radiographs occupy the whole of the depth of the mandible, usually have a sturdy lingual plate which adequately maintains the continuity of the bone through the operation.

The relationship of the cyst to adjacent structures is more important. Vital teeth which have a satisfactory periodontal condition and are functional, should be preserved. Consideration should be given to retaining dead teeth in well-cared-for mouths. This may be done by root-filling and apicectomy providing that at the very least the whole of the coronal half of the root is firmly held in sound alveolar bone. Dead teeth should be extracted where they are non-functional, mobile, the periodontal condition is poor, the patient already wears a denture. Where a diagnosis of keratocyst has been confirmed, extraction of involved teeth may be wise to ensure removal of all the lining in view of the high reported recurrence rate.

Dentigerous cysts contain teeth and, in the young where these are reasonably well placed, treatment may be directed to saving the tooth and allowing it to erupt into the arch.

Cysts may be closely related to the maxillary sinus, floor of nose or to the inferior dental canal, which are important structures not to be damaged and may modify the treatment plan. The maxillary antrum can be partially of even completely obliterated by a large cyst. In the mandible the inferior dental nerve may be grossly displaced in a similar way.

Treatment

Acutely infected cysts are treated with antibacterial drugs and by drainage; further surgery is delayed till the acute phase has settled. There are two methods for treating cysts, enucleation and marsupialisation.

Enucleation

In this operation the whole of the cyst lining is removed. For this reason, and because healing proceeds more rapidly after this has been done, it is the best treatment, particularly for keratocysts, and should be used whenever possible. Though applicable to all types of cyst it is seldom necessary in treating cysts of eruption and is contraindicated in dentigerous cysts if the enclosed tooth is to be preserved.

Small apical cysts where the tooth is to be retained (apicectomy). The tooth should have a conventional root filling just before surgery unless this is mechanically

Fig. 64 Apicectomy. Left: Apicetomy flap – dotted line shows proposed level of section of root. *Right:* after root section. Note root cut level with bone margin. Saucerisation may be completed by removing buccal plate to level of dotted line.

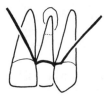
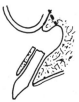

impossible. The incision is made round the neck of the affected tooth with two vertical incisions diverging into the buccal sulcus. The flap is then reflected to expose the bone over the apex (Fig. 64).

The position of the root in the alveolar bone is estimated and the apical third exposed. This may be done with a medium-sized rosehead bur. Bone is then removed to expose the cystic area, taking care to avoid damaging, or even exposing, the roots of neighbouring teeth. The apical third of the root is divided using a No. 5 fissure bur. The anterior part of the root should be cut flush with the alveolar bone. (Fig. 64).

The cyst lining is then enucleated. This does not mean curettage, but implies a careful, methodical separation of the cyst from bone to remove the lining intact without tearing if possible. Curettes (Mitchell's trimmer) can be used, if kept well against bone, to dissect out the cyst gently (Fig. 65). Where the lining is firmly attached, 1.5 cm ribbon gauze soaked in saline or in diluted hydrogen peroxide may be packed carefully into the cavity to separate the two tissues (Fig. 65). The lining is sent for histological examination. The cavity is examined for any remnants of granulations or cyst lining. These are frequently far back behind the root of the tooth and are removed by scraping the bony walls; none must be left if a recurrence is to be avoided. Where the tooth has been root filled the apical seal is checked. Should this be inadequate a retrograde filling is placed in the apex. The cavity is thoroughly washed out and the flap replaced and sutured.

Where a prosthetic crown is present it is unwise to incise around the gingival margin and a semi-lunar incision 3 cm long is made with its lowest point at least 0.5 cm above the gingival margin. Care must be taken when removing bone to ensure that at the end of the operation the flap margin is adequately supported on bone.

Enucleation of the larger odontogenic cysts. The chief problems in the treatment of large cysts by enucleation are to provide a flap which will give adequate

Fig. 65 Enucleation of cyst. (*a*) Curette used to enucleate cyst with the back of the spoon turned towards cyst lining. (*b*) At greatest diameter of cyst the curette is reversed to present concavity of spoon to the cyst lining. (*c*) Packing wet ribbon gauze between cyst lining and bone to separate them.

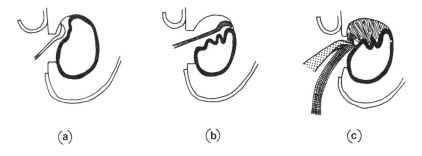

(a)   (b)   (c)

closure and to establish the maximum amount of clot that will organise without liquefying or becoming infected. When these objects are achieved the cyst will heal by first intention with minimal deformity.

Flap. The incision is made at the *cervical margin of the teeth* or along the alveolar crest in edentulous patients. It should be twice the length of the cyst and, if possible, of equal length on each side of its centre. As the flap is to be transported the vertical incisions are made so that *the base is shorter than the free margin*. This unusual design is only satisfactory because the blood supply is adequate due to the great length of the flap in relation to its width (Fig. 66). Where the bone resorption has brought cyst lining and mucoperiosteum into apposition the two should be separated without tearing either, and the flap reflected beyond the cyst lining on to bone. This is usually the most difficult part of the operation.

Enucleation. The whole of the cyst lining must be enucleated. After its removal it is carefully examined for any tears or deficiencies. Only where it is intact can the dental surgeon be sure no lining has been left behind. The cavity is systematically searched and any soft tissue remnants curetted out. This is particularly important where a keratocyst is suspected. The bone edges are saucerised to provide a smooth transition from cyst cavity to the surface of the bone (Fig. 66). Saucerisation can be extensive providing that the alveolar crest is preserved to leave a satisfactory ridge for dentures and that vital structures are not damaged. Anteriorly the bony support to the ala of the nose must not be undermined lest an ugly deformity occur.

Closure. The two ends of the flap are transposed towards the centre of the cyst to provide tissue which will fall into the saucerised cavity when the

Fig. 66 Enucleation of large dental cysts. (*a*) Design of flap (note vertical incisions). (*b*) Flap replaced; the deficiency over the bone is shaded. (*c*) Section of cyst cavity before saucerisation. (*d*) After saucerisation. (*e*) Flap replaced. (*f*) Pack placed over *mucosal flap* and lip sutured to alveolar crest through both edges of wound.

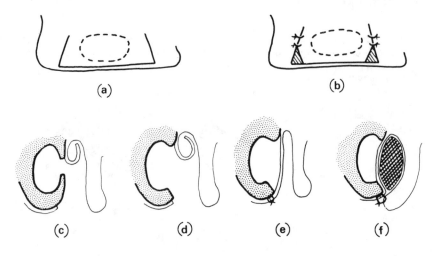

(a)　　(b)

(c)　　(d)　　(e)　　(f)

free margin is sutured back to the alveolar crest. The first suture is put at the centre of the flap and the remainder are so placed as to pucker it slightly. Apposition to bone is only attempted at the cavity margins. The blood clot in the dead space is reduced and sealed in by making the flap follow the contour of the saucer. For the clot to organise without breaking down it must be a thin layer into which granulations from bone and soft tissue can grow rapidly, so post-operative bleeding, with consequent bulging of the flap, must be prevented. This achieved by placing a gauze pack in the buccal sulcus *over the flap* in the area of saucerisation. It is held in place by suturing cheek or lip to the alveolar crest so that there is contact between buccal and alveolar mucous membrane. This also assists in maintaining a satisfactory buccal sulcus (Fig. 66). Added support may be given by an external pressure dressing. Both packs may be removed after forty-eight hours or when post-operative haemorrhage has ceased. Alternatively, the clot may be reduced by adequate drainage. For cysts in the mandible a drain can be placed from the cavity through the lingual wall below the floor of the mouth and brought out onto the skin of the neck. The drain is removed after forty-eight hours.

Various substances have been packed into the cyst cavity to obliterate the dead space. Fibrin foam and gelatine sponge *only form a matrix* for a large clot which may still become infected. The use of bone is more rational and chips have been successfully employed, but also carry a risk of infection. Rarely, in very large cysts of the mandible, the bone can be so weakened at operation that it may be necessary to place an immediate bone graft in the cavity.

Marsupialisation

An opening into the cyst is made so that the contents drain out and the lining epithelium is exposed to the mouth. Its advantages are simplicity, speed of operation, minimal trauma and that no bone is exposed to contamination from the mouth. This makes it ideal for ill patients unable to undergo a long procedure or a general anaesthetic. Marsupialisation lessens the danger of damaging vital structures, the alveolar ridge is preserved and indeed, if properly planned, the operation may improve the depth of the buccal sulcus and the retention of dentures, particularly in the lower jaw. It has two major disadvantages: pathological tissues are left and healing is slow. It should be the treatment of choice only for eruption cysts and dentigerous cysts where the tooth is to be preserved. In large cysts where the jaw may fracture or vital structures, particularly teeth, could be damaged by enucleation, marsupialisation may be used as a first procedure. Once bone has reformed the remaining lining is enucleated at a second operation. This technique has also been successfully used for large keratocysts of the ascending ramus where because the lining is in contact with periosteum over a wide area and dissection is difficult there is a danger of seeding into the soft tissues. Even in this group of cysts new bone appears to reform and make later enucleation safe.

Operation.   A buccal incision is made along the occlusal margin of the cyst and curved at each end to follow its contour in the bone. The flap should be large. Some operators make a small hole which tends to close and requires packing over a long period because a satisfactory obturator cannot be fitted. It must be accepted that where many natural teeth are present only a small opening can be made.

The flap is then reflected and the bone removed as widely as possible over the cyst. A window which closely follows the bone margins is cut in the lining with scissors. This tissue should be sent for histological examination. The mucosal flap is now excised so that cyst lining and mucosa can be sewn together round the edges of the window (Fig. 67). The cavity is washed out and temporarily dressed with Whitehead's varnish or Bismuth, Iodoform Paraffin Paste (B.I.P.P.) on ribbon gauze. With a large window in an edentulous area the pack and sutures may be removed after ten days and an obturator constructed on a denture. The patient is given a water syringe to keep the cavity clean. As the cavity obliterates the obturator will require reduction. Where the aperture is small and an obturator cannot be worn, packing must continue until healing is complete. In dentigerous cysts containing an erupting tooth the same procedure is followed, care being taken not to disturb the tooth.

Marsupialisation into the antrum.   Large cysts which encroach on the maxillary antrum can be marsupialised into it. This avoids a gross deformity in the

Fig. 67   Marsupialisation. (a) The pre-operative outline of cyst in mandible. (b) Black line shows line of incision in buccal mucoperiosteum and following the outline of the cyst (dotted line). (c) Removal of buccal bone to expose cyst but preserve the alveolar ridge. (d) Cyst opened, drained, and lining sutured to mucous membrane.

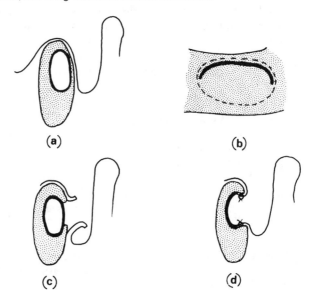

(a)

(b)

(c)

(d)

buccal sulcus which may take a long time to heal. The cyst is exposed as for enucleation and a window cut in the lining. Through this a direct opening into the antrum is made where cyst and antrum lining are in apposition. This should be as large as possible and never less than 2.5 cm across. This technique may be combined with enucleation of cysts which are adherent only to the antrum lining. The operation can also be performed through a Caldwell-Luc approach into the antrum when a hole is cut from the antrum into the cyst.

Combined enucleation and open packing. Large cysts can be enucleated, but instead of an immediate closure the mucosal flap is turned into the cavity to cover some of the raw bone and a pack is inserted to protect the rest. This technique overcomes the risk of breakdown of the blood clot present in immediate closure. As the pathological lining has all been removed, healing is far faster than when the cavity is marsupialised.

Follow-up

Long-term follow-up of all cysts is advisable lest retained epithelial fragments cause a recurrence. Satisfactory healing can be assessed by clinical examination, and by radiopaque lamina round the periphery of the cyst and new bone formation filling the radiolucent area.

Keratocysts may recur a long time after operation; follow-up of these lesions must continue over a long period of years.

Developmental cysts of non-dental origin

Inclusion or fissural cysts of the jaws

These arise from the inclusion of epithelial remnants at the site of fusion of the various processes that form the mouth and face. They are epithelial lined and usually contain mucoid fluid. As they do not arise from the teeth, vitality testing is essential in the differential diagnosis.

Nasolabial cysts

They occur at the junction of the globular, lateral and median nasal processes, under the ala of the nose. They are diagnosed by their position as they lie in a depression on the maxilla, and not in the bone.

Median cysts

These very rare cysts are found in the midline where fusion of the two halves of the palate and mandible takes place.

Incisive canal cysts

These develop from epithelial remnants in the incisive canal. They present as a swelling under the incisive papilla which, on an anterior occlusal radiograph, shows as an expansion of the incisive foramen. The latter is normally under 7 mm in diameter. Occasionally the presenting symptom is a complaint of a salty taste.

Globulomaxillary cysts

These occur at the junction of the globular and maxillary processes. They arise between the maxillary lateral incisor and canine, characteristically separating the roots of these teeth which are not concerned with the formation of the cyst and should be vital.

Diagnosis and assessment. This is approached in the same way as for cysts of dental origin and the differential diagnosis is made by their special features. These are their site, fluid contents, and the fact that adjacent teeth are vital because the cysts are of non-dental origin.

Treatment. They are treated like other cysts of the jaws by enucleation or by marsupialisation followed by enucleation where there is risk of damaging adjacent teeth.

Dermoid cysts. These arise from inclusion of ectoderm at lines of fusion anywhere in the body. In the mouth they may be found in the floor, the palate, or the tongue. They are teratomas lined by stratified squamous epithelium and may contain hair, nails, teeth etc.

Diagnosis. Those in the floor of the mouth may occur in the midline or laterally. They do not become obvious until adolescence or later. The patient complains of a slowly enlarging swelling under the tongue, occasionally affecting speech, and which is visible in the neck. Examination reveals a fluctuant or soft swelling in the floor of the mouth either above or below the mylohyoid. It does not move up or down on swallowing, which is important in distinguishing it from a thyroglossal cyst, Aspiration produces a thick sebaceous material, where this can be withdrawn. Dermoid cysts at other sites are similarly diagnosed.

Treatment. Sublingual dermoids may be enucleated through an external approach below the mandible or intraorally through an incision in the floor of the mouth, just at the reflection of the lingual mucosa from the mandible. The latter flap is reflected lingually and will contain the ducts of the submandibular glands which must not be damaged. The cyst is then exposed but may have to be emptied to remove it as otherwise it may be too large to pass out of the incision. Its thick lining makes it easy to enucleate. Satisfactory drainage must be provided for a few days for the large sublingual deficiency.

Retention cysts

These are discussed under diseases of the salivary glands (Chapter XVI).

Further reading

Browne, R. M. (1975), 'The pathogenesis of odotogenic cysts', *J. Oral Path.*, **4**, 31.

Killer, H. C., Kay, L. W. and Seward, G. R. (1977), *Benign Cystic Lesions of the Jaws*, 3rd edn. Churchill Livingstone, Edinburgh.

Seward, G. R., Harris, M. and McGowan, D. A. (1987). *Killey and Kay's Outline of Oral Surgery*, 2nd edn. John Wright, Bristol.

Shafer, W. G., Hine, M. K. and Levy, B. M. (1983). *A textbook of Oral Pathology*, 4th edn. W. B. Sanders, Philadelphia.

xiv Treatment of fractured jaws

The commonest causes of fractured jaws are road traffic accidents, fights, falls and sport. They occur chiefly in males between fifteen and thirty five years of age and twice as frequently in the mandible as in the maxilla. Fractures may be direct, following a blow at the point where the break occurs, or may be indirect as a result of a blow on the bone at some distance from where the lesion occurs. They may be single linear or comminuted, that is fragmented into one or more small pieces, and are said to be compound when they communicate with a wound of the skin or mucous membrane. Where there is a tooth in the line of the fracture the latter is almost certainly compound into the mouth through the periodontal membrane. In the young, incomplete or greenstick fractures of the mandible can occur. Diseases of the bone predispose to spontaneous pathological fractures.

Applied anatomy

For describing injuries the face is divided into three parts. The lower third is the mandible and the soft tissues covering it. The middle third is bounded below by the occlusal line of the maxillary teeth and above by a line drawn through the pupils. The upper third lies above this, but is not the province of the dental surgeon.

The mandible

The commonest sites of fracture in the mandible are the condyle neck, the angle and the canine region. The condyle may fracture through its thin neck either within the capsule or below it, and may be bilateral as a result of blows to the chin, particularly if the mouth is open, or unilateral following blows to the body of the mandible on the opposite side. Fractures of the coronoid process are uncommon.

The angle of the mandible is a weak point because there is a change in direction of the grain of the bone which occurs where the vertical ascending ramus and horizontal body meet. Further, the shape of the mandible in cross-section changes as the thick lower border of the body becomes thin at the angle, so that the lower third molar tooth sits in bone with little basal support lingually. Finally, the third molar, particularly if it is unerupted, may occupy up to two-thirds of the depth of the bone.

The body is the strongest part of the lower jaw but is weakened by the presence of the tooth sockets. The canine has a long, broad root and its socket is a common site of fracture. The symphysis may also be involved as a result of blows on the chin. Alveolar fractures occur chiefly in the incisor region.

Displacement.   Displacement depends on three factors, the force of the blow, gravity and the pull of the muscles inserted into the bone. The muscles concerned are the suprahyoid group attached to the lingual aspect of the anterior part of the mandible which depress the lower jaw, and the muscles of mastication (masseter, temporalis and medial pterygoid) inserted into the ascending ramus which elevate the mandible and move it laterally. The lateral pterygoid muscle, inserted into the condyle and meniscus of the temporomandibular joint, draws the condyle forward and therefore assists in opening the mouth.

Condylar fractures.   In these cases the lateral pterygoid muscle draws the fractured head forward medially and, in certain cases, over the eminentia articularis and out of the glenoid fossa to produce a fracture dislocation. The other muscles of mastication raise the ramus of the affected side to produce an anterior open bite between the incisors and canines on the *opposite side.* On opening the mouth the body of the mandible is displaced towards the affected side with marked deviation of the midline. In bilateral condylar fractures both ascending rami are drawn up and back equally so that gagging occurs on the posterior teeth causing an anterior open bite on both sides.

Fractures of the angle or body.   In these the suprahyoid group of muscles depress the anterior part of the mandible. Posteriorly the pull of the muscles of mastication attached to the ascending ramus draw it upwards. The posterior fragment is also drawn inwards as the pull of the medial pterygoid muscle is stronger than that of the masseter (Fig. 68). Displacement is resisted by the periosteum, if it is intact, by the occlusion of the teeth, and by the impaction of the fractured bone ends against each other. This last depends on the angle of the line of fracture which is said to be *unfavourable* if it would allow the posterior fragment to displace or *favourable* if it prevents it doing so.

Fig. 68   Effects of muscle pull on mandibular fractures. Arrows indicate the direction of muscle pull. (a) Horizontal view of mandible showing horizontaly favourable fracture (dotted line) and horizontally unfavourable fracture (continuous line), (b) Vertical view showing vertically favourable (dotted line) and unfavourable (continuous line) fractures.

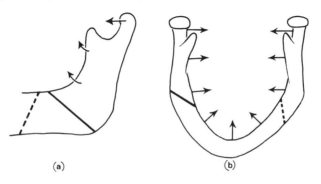

(a)   (b)

As displacement can take place in two planes, upwards and inwards, fractures are described as favourable or unfavourable when viewed from *the side or horizontally*, and from *above or vertically*. Thus a *horizontally unfavourable fracture displaces upwards, a vertically unfavourable fracture inwards* (Fig. 68).

Where a bilateral fracture occurs in the anterior region through the canine sockets it is possible for the geniohyoid, genioglossus and mylohyoid muscles to displace the loose anterior portion downwards and backwards, with loss of control of the tongue which may fall back into the pharynx and obstruct the airway.

Midline fracture. In oblique fractures through the symphysis of the mandible, one half may be displaced lingually by the mylohyoid muscle to cause over-riding in the midline.

Age. In children the mandible is greatly weakened by the numerous crypts of the developing teeth but the greater elasticity of the bone compensates for this. In older patients the bones get more brittle and tend to break more easily and the mandible is weakened by resorption of the alveolar bone after the teeth are lost. The periosteum does however form a complete envelope round the edentulous mandible which, if not torn in the accident, holds the fractured ends in apposition. With advancing years the mandible becomes more dependent for its blood supply on the periosteum than on the inferior dental artery. For this reason methods of reduction or fixation which involve stripping of the periosteum must be avoided in the elderly.

Middle third of the face

Fractures of the middle third of the face involve a complex of bones which include the paired bones, the maxilla, palatine, zygomatic, nasal, lachrymal and inferior conchae, together with the single vomer and ethmoid bones. The structure of the maxillary complex consists of strong vertical buttresses, the chief of which are formed by the frontal process of the maxilla, the zygomatic process of the maxilla with the zygomatic bone, and the pterygoid plates of the sphenoid with the tuberosity of the maxilla. The spaces between the buttresses are closed by thin bone plates which enclose several large cavities, the maxillary air sinuses, the nasal cavity, and the orbits. The base of the complex is strengthened by the alveolar bone and the palate. This construction offers great resistance to upward forces such as occur in mastication, but very little to shearing stress from a horizontal blow.

Classification of maxillary fractures. Fractures of the middle third of the face fall into five categories (Fig. 69). Those of the alveolus which occur in the anterior region from a blow or in the tuberosity during tooth extraction. Those where the palate and alveolar process are separated from the maxillary complex by a transverse fracture just above the floor of the antrum and of the nose, called Guerin's or Le Fort I fractures. In the third group the fracture line passes through the lateral and anterior walls of both maxillary sinuses and continues up through the infraorbital ridges to join across the bridge of the nose (Fig. 69). This is known as a pyramidal or

Fig. 69 Fractures of maxilla. *A*, Alveolar fracture. *B*, Le Fort I or Guerin's fracture. *C*, dashed line, Le Fort II. *D*, dotted line, Le Fort III.

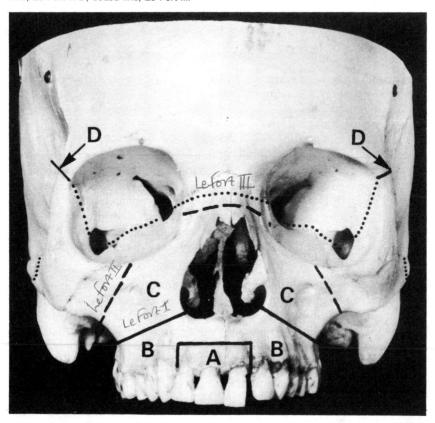

Le Fort II fracture. In the fourth category the maxillary complex is virtually separated from the cranium by a fracture which traverses the lateral wall of both orbits, both orbital floors, and crosses the midline at the root of the nose to involve the cribiform plate of the ethmoid. This is named a high transverse or Le Fort III. The clinical importance of this classification is that the Le Fort I involves only the palate and the maxillary antrum. The Le Fort II involves the antrum, floor of the orbit and the nose. The Le Fort III includes the structures affected by Le Fort II and also the anterior cranial fossa. Finally, the malar bone can be fractured by a direct blow which may drive in the prominence of the cheek. The fracture line passes through the infraorbital ridge, the anterior wall of the antrum, the malar buttress, the zygomatic arch and the frontal process of the zygoma. Many combinations of these fractures do occur.

Displacement. In maxillary fractures the displacement is caused by the force of the blow and not by muscle pull as none of the muscles attached to the maxilla are strong enough to move the fragments. The most usual displacement is backwards and downwards, causing a typical concavity of the face (dish-face) with anterior open bite due to gagging on the posterior teeth. This open bite is particularly marked in the Guerin's type fracture.

Diagnosis

The dental surgeon should proceed to make a diagnosis in the usual way unless some urgent condition, such as asphyxia or haemorrhage, requires immediate attention.

History

The time of the accident is important in assessing the urgency of treatment, and the degree of infection in compound fractures. The difficulty of reducing misplaced fractures increases as healing progresses. A history of any previous facial injury is important as old injuries can occasionally cause confusion in the diagnosis. The patient's general condition and any tenderness or bruising of the head, chest or abdomen are noted. Shock is unusual in facial injuries and, unless the blood loss has been excessive, the cause should be sought elsewhere.

The patient should be asked if he was knocked out. In unconscious or confused patients causes other than concussion such as alcohol, insulin or diabetic coma, or a cardiovascular catastrophe should be considered. Any drug administered previously, especially sedatives, analgesics or antibacterials, should be recorded in the notes.

Examination

The surgeon must look for the following signs of a fracture. *Swelling and bruising* are usual at the point where the patient was struck, but may not coincide with the site of an indirect fracture. *Deformity* of the bone contour can be masked by swelling, but examination may reveal a break in the continuity of the bone or displacement. Intraorally *derangement of the occlusion* may localise the fracture. *Abnormal movement* in the bone is diagnostic, and when it occurs may be accompanied by *pain* and by *crepitus* or grating as the rough bone ends rub against each other. *Loss of function* in the jaws is common as a result of *trismus* or pain. The function of nerves, muscles and of the eyes may all be affected in fractures.

The facial bones are most conveniently examined in the dental chair. Should the patient be too ill to get out of bed the headboard may be removed to allow access from the head of the bed.

Extraoral. The patient is first looked at full face for obvious signs of injury. Lacerations should not be probed or touched but are immediately covered with a dressing. Clots present in the nose and ears should not be disturbed but a discharge of cerebrospinal fluid from these orifices is an important finding indicating a fracture of the cranial base. To distinguish it from nasal secretion it should be tested for glucose, a constituent of cerebrospinal fluid.

The surgeon should then move behind the patient and, looking down from above, he uses the tips of his fingers to palpate and compare the right and left sides, and to determine points of tenderness or breaks in the continuity of the facial bones. He starts with the superior, lateral and inferior margins of the orbit and then proceeds to the bridge of the nose, where any deviation from the midline or depression is noted. The malar prominences are compared to detect loss of contour. Where there is marked oedema it may be very difficult to do this with certainty, but firm steady pressure on the swelling for a few moments will push it away and allow the bone to be felt.

The fingers then move over the zygomatic arch, to the temporomandibular joints. The patient is asked to open and close the mouth and perform lateral movements. The range of opening and of lateral movement is assessed. Fractures of the zygomatic arch may prevent opening as the coronoid process may jam against the displaced zygomatic process. In fractures of the condyle or ascending ramus there is little movement of the condyle head on the affected side or the mandible towards the opposite side. When the joint is difficult to palpate the little finger may be put into the external auditory meatus and the condyle felt through the anterior wall. Palpation is then continued to compare the ascending ramus, the angles and the lower border of the body of the mandible.

The surgeon then moves to face the patient and examines the eyes for damage, particularly depression, proptosis or a difference in level. Subconjunctival haemorrhage in the upper half of the eye suggests bleeding from a fracture of the roof of the orbit, and in the lower part of the conjunctiva a fracture of the orbital floor, but in severe injuries the whole of the conjunctiva may be involved. Each eye is checked individually for vision and then both together for movement vertically and horizontally and for double vision (diplopia) in all fields. This can be done by moving a finger up, down and across where it can be clearly seen by both eyes at once. Abnormalities of movement and diplopia may be due to paralysis of the extrinsic muscles of the eye as a result of cranial injury. Diplopia alone may be caused by detachment of the suspensory ligament in malar or maxillary fractures, herniation of orbital fat through defects in the orbital floor or by oedema, all of which may alter the position of the eyeball. Oedema can also mask diplopia by compensating for a fall in level which may only become apparent when the swelling recedes. The examination concludes with tests for loss of sensation in the branches of the trigeminal nerve, particularly the infraorbital, which is affected in malar and maxillary fractures, and the mental nerve involved in mandibular injuries. Function of the facial nerve is checked by asking the patient to move his forehead, eyelids and lips.

Intraoral. The lips are gently parted and the mucosa, floor of the mouth and tongue examined for lacerations or haematoma. A haematoma of the floor of the mouth is a sign of a fracture of the mandible. The teeth are charted and those that are lost, grossly carious or fractured are noted, together with any disturbance of the occlusion. Where teeth (or denture fragments) are missing and cannot be accounted for, particularly if the patient has lost consciousness, the chest should be radiographed. Percussion of the teeth may give a 'cracked teacup' note suggestive of a broken tooth or of a fractured jaw, particularly in the maxilla. The upper buccal sulcus is palpated for any sharp edges of bone or bruising diagnostic of a fracture through the malar buttress.

Fractures of the maxillary alveolus or a midline split of the palate are detected by grasping the alveolar segments and trying gently at first to move them buccally or compress them lingually. The maxillary complex is then tested by grasping the alveolus and the teeth in one hand and trying to elicit movement, whilst the other hand palpates extraorally to determine the level at which the fracture has occurred. The fingers are placed in turn over the root of the nose, at the infraorbital margins and in the canine fossa.

Similarly the mandible is grasped in both hands, with the fingers over the occlusal surface of the teeth and the thumbs under the lower border, and tested in segments for mobility. The clinical findings should be written down and a provisional diagnosis made before radiographs are ordered.

Diagnosis

Λ summary of the diagnostic features of various fractures is shown in Table 7.

Radiographs

These are taken to establish the presence of fractures, the direction in which they run and the amount by which they are displaced, and to identify radiopaque foreign bodies such as glass in the soft tissues. Medicolegally they are considered a diagnostic measure of the first importance. They also provide a visual record of the progress of the patient.

Radiographs of all fractures must be taken in two planes. The following views usually give a satisfactory survey of the facial bones, and wherever there is doubt about the extent of the injuries all five should be taken. They are a right and left 30° lateral oblique view of the mandible, a posteroanterior view of the mandible, occipitomental view of the sinuses, and a true lateral of the facial bones. The midline of the mandible is difficult to see except on an occlusal film. Where available and the patient ambulatory the orthopantomograph can replace the lateral oblique views. Examination of the radiographs is first made to identify all the normal structures and the bony margins of the facial bones. Both sides of the jaws are compared for differences on the outline. It is important to recognise shadows thrown by such normal structures as the oropharyngeal airway, hyoid bone or intervertebral spaces which may simulate fractures in certain projections.

The 30° lateral oblique view of the mandible. This covers the mandible from the premolar region to the ascending ramus and sometimes the neck of the condyle (Fig. 70). As it is taken in the horizontal plane it will demonstrate fractures which are horizontally favourable or unfavourable, the latter may be displaced upwards. A rotated 30° lateral oblique will show the premolar and canine region better.

Table 7 All these signs and symptoms are not found in every case. Radiographs will show a lack of continuity in the bone at the site of the fracture.

Site	Signs and symptoms	
Unilateral condyle	Affected side:	Pain in joint, worse on moving Tenderness and swelling Absence (or abnormality) of movements of condyle head Deviation of mandible towards this side Gagging on molar teeth
		Opposite side: open bite Limitation of lateral excursion to that side
Bilateral condyle	Pain, tenderness and swelling over both joints Gagging on the posterior teeth and an anterior open bite Restricted lateral movements Absence of movement of condyle heads	
Body of the mandible	Pain on moving jaw Trismus Movement and crepitus at site of fracture Step deformity of lower border of mandible Derangement of the occlusion Mental anaesthesia Haematoma in the floor of mouth and buccal mucosa	
Malar	Depression of the prominence of the cheek Step deformity in the infraorbital ridge Subconjunctival haemorrhage and diplopia Infraorbital nerve anaesthesia Haematoma intraorally over the malar buttress Blood in the antrum Trismus due to the coronoid process impacting against the displaced malar or zygomatic arch Circumorbital ecchymosis	
Guerin's (Le Fort I)	Floating palate Blood in the antrum Bilateral haematoma in buccal sulcus Deranged occlusion with anterior open bite	
Low pyramidal (Le Fort II)	Gross swelling and, after oedema subsides, dish-faced deformity Subconjunctival haemorrhage and diplopia Bilateral infraorbital nerve anaesthesia Bilateral haematoma intraorally over malar buttresses Retroposed upper dental arch with anterior open bite	
High transverse (Le Fort III)	Gross swelling and, after oedema, subsides, dish-faced deformity Subconjunctival haemorrhage and sometimes diplopia Retroposed upper dental arch with anterior open bite Cerebrospinal fluid leak from nose Signs of head injury	

Fig. 70 Lateral oblique view of mandible showing upward displacement of distal fragment in horizontally unfavourable fracture. Drawing (a) shows how one oblique fracture passing through inner and outer cortical plates may give a false appearance of a double fracture on radiograph. (b) In such a case the fracture lines are always seen to meet at the upper and lower border of the bone.

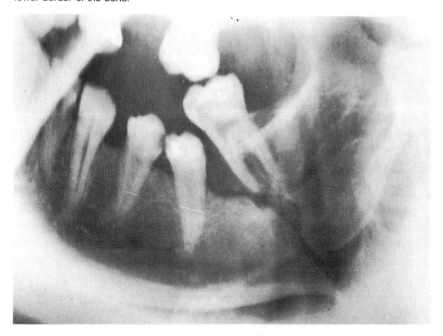

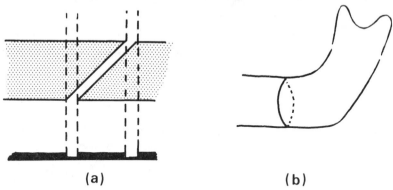

(a)   (b)

The orthopantomograph. This tomographic radiograph of the jaws may replace the lateral oblique views. The mandible from condyle to condyle is seen but due to superimposition of the cervical spine the canine and incisor regions are not well visualised. As the rotation of the X-ray tube changes direction in the premolar region caution is needed in interpretation of the film in this area. It is unsuitable for any patient who is unable to stand or sit whilst the radiograph is being taken.

The postero-anterior view of the mandible. The whole of the mandible from the condyle neck to the midline on both sides is shown. As the rays pass through the angle of the mandible from the lower border to the occlusal surface they give a vertical view of this area and allow vertically favourable and unfavourable fractures to be assessed (Fig. 71).

Fig. 71 Posterior-anterior view of mandible showing a vertically favourable fracture through the angle on the left. Drawing shows how a vertically unfavourable fracture (*VU*) may not show on this view as the break in continuity of the cortical plates may not be projected on the radiograph. A vertically favourable fracture (*VF*) is usually clearly seen.

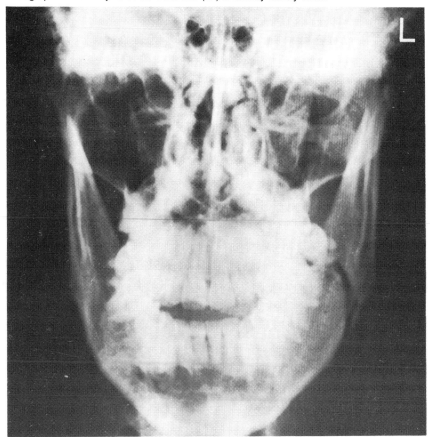

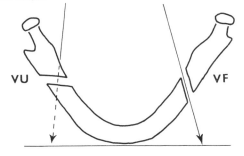

The occipitomental view. This is examined in a series of transverse sweeps following the bony contours at the levels of the supraorbital ridges, of the infraorbital margins, and the zygomatic arch, of the antral wall, nasal wall and vomer, and finally the level of the mandibular/maxillary occlusion and of the lower border of the mandible. It demonstrates fractures of the maxillary complex, and radiopacity of the maxillary sinus which may be the result of bleeding into the antrum from a fracture of one of its walls (Fig. 72). Fifteen- or thirty-degree occipito-mental and stereoscopic occipito-mental views are both of assistance in detecting displacement not shown on the standard view. Fractures of the zygomatic arch are best shown on a submento-vertical film.

True lateral of facial bones. This shows separation of the maxilla from the cranial base, or of the palate from the maxilla.

Fig. 72 Occipito-mental radiograph showing fractures of middle third of face.

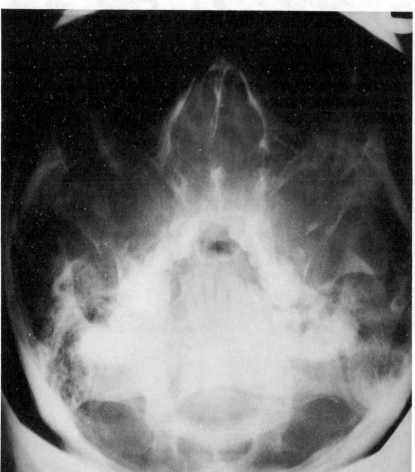

Other radiographs of importance are occlusal films and intraoral apical views of the teeth showing their relationship to the fracture line or fracture of their roots. Special views of the temporomandibular joints may be necessary to show the condyles and the condyle neck.

Study models

Frequently the patient is unable to bring his teeth into occlusion or the fractures are badly comminuted so that the normal relationship of the teeth can only be seen on study models.

Treatment planning

The aims of treatment are to restore function and to achieve a good aesthetic result, but treatment must be modified according to the patient's general condition. The only immediate local measures required are attention to the airway, arrest of haemorrhage and control of infection. Where multiple injuries are present the dental surgeon is responsible for explaining the degree of urgency for treatment of the jaws to achieve a satisfactory result. Thereafter, planning is done jointly with the other specialists involved. It is generally agreed that bony injuries heal better the earlier they are treated but, in the presence of gross oedema or large haematomas, they are best left a few days for these to settle.

Emergency care

Airway. In unconscious patients respiratory obstruction may be caused by blood clot, or a foreign body in the oropharynx or larynx. In bilateral fractures of the mandible through the canine region the tongue may fall helplessly back to occlude the airway. In maxillary injuries the palate can be displaced down and back to occlude the pharynx.

Treatment is urgent. The tongue or palate is drawn forward and the mouth and pharynx sucked or wiped clear of debris to re-establish the airway. To keep the tongue forward, a suture may be passed through it, or the patient turned face down which also allows saliva and blood to drain out of the mouth. Where these measures are ineffective an emergency tracheostomy may be necessary. Before giving an anaesthetic soon after the accident the stomach must be emptied of swallowed blood using a Ryle's tube.

Haemorrhage. Acute bleeding, though seldom of long duration, is controlled as described in Chapter VII. Reduction and fixation will often arrest haemorrhage because movement disturbs the natural arrest. The pulse and blood pressure should be monitored to ensure that the patient does not become shocked.

Prevention of infection. External wounds are kept covered with dressings and a prophylactic course of an antibacterial drug administered. They should be closed as soon as possible, under local anaesthesia if necessary.

Pain. This surprisingly, is seldom severe, particularly if open wounds are covered and some form of temporary support has been provided. Morphine or its derivaties must not be given because they may mask the signs of increasing intracranial pressure, or depress the patient with an embarrassed airway. Soluble distalgesic tablets may be prescribed.

Temporary immobilisation. This can be provided by a bandage, but careful consideration must be given to the effect this may have on the fragments. An ill-applied bandage may increase the displacement, and backward pressure on a bilateral fracture of the mandible can displace the tongue back into the pharynx. Many temporary supports are used; the best are probably the barrel bandage (Fig. 73) and the elastic chin bandage attached to a headcap.

Supportive treatment. This has been discussed in Chapters II and IV

Head injury. Many patients who sustain facial injuries may also have been concussed. All these patients, however short the time they were unconscious, must be under the care of a neurosurgeon and carefully observed. The diagnosis of head injury depends on a comparison of signs and symptoms over a period and because the dental surgeon may be the first to see them he should record the following. Headache and vomiting is noted. The level of consciousness is important. The conscious patient may be rational or confused: if unconscious and in semi-coma he will respond to pricking of the limbs, whereas the deeply comatose subject will not. Movements of the limbs should be noted and whether they are normal or abnormal. The eyes should be examined and the pupil reactions tested. A rise in intracranial pressure is denoted by a slow reaction to light of the pupil on the affected side and with increasing pressure it becomes fixed and dilated. In the final stage the opposite pupil is also dilated. In all head injuries the pupils should be tested at intervals and any abnormality in reaction regarded as a matter of urgency.

Finally it is wise to institute a half-hourly record of pulse, blood pressure and pupil reaction to light, as these reflect changes in intracranial pressure.

It is stressed that the dental surgeon's object in making these simple observations is to provide records that will assist his surgical colleague in diagnosis and treatment.

It is emphasised that all Le Fort III fractures are head injuries and should be monitored as such. Further as the anterior cranial fossa communicates with the nose through the fractured cribriform plate there is grave danger of an ascending infection. The patient must be protected from a meningeal infection by an antibacterial drug which will cross the thecal barrier, the drug of choice being sulphadimidine. Where, after reduction and immobilisation of the facial fractures, a cerebrospinal fluid leak persists, intercranial repair of the dura may be advised by neurosurgeons.

Fig. 73 Barrel bandage. *Left:* crepe bandage passed under mandible and tied in a simple knot. *Right:* knot opened to go round the patient's head. *Below:* tails tied on top of the head, bandage not over point of chin.

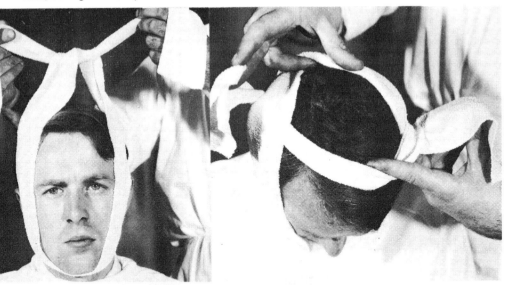

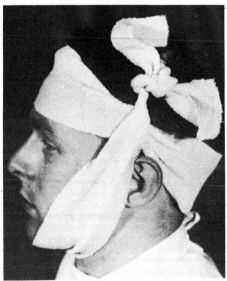

Natural repair of bone

The healing of fractures takes place entirely by the natural process of bone repair. Treatment is directed to providing ideal conditions for this to take place.

Between the fractured ends of the bone a blood clot forms. Within four days capillaries, fibroblasts and inflammatory cells invade this and begin replacing it with granulation tissue. Along the bony margins of the fracture osteoclasts appear which resorb the bone; this is seen on radiographs as a widening of the fracture line. Osteoblasts from the periosteum and cancellous bone invade the granulations and lay down a collagenous matrix called osteoid. The acidity of the tissues caused by the initial inflammatory reaction subsidies after ten days and this allows calcification to proceed. Bony union takes place in four to six weeks.

The pattern of the new bone or callus is at first irregular but later, over a period of about six months in the mandible, reorganisation to normal bone structure takes place. In long bones an excess of callus is formed round the bone ends, and its presence on radiographs is accepted as a sign that satisfactory union is proceeding. This does not happen in the mandible, where formation of callus is usually limited to the space between the bone ends and therefore shows little on radiographs. Maxillary fractures may heal by fibrous union only.

Principles of treatment

The aim of treatment is to restore function, which is the first consideration, and to achieve a good aesthetic result.

Control of infection

Repair, particularly new bone formation, cannot take place in the presence of infection. To prevent this occurring all foreign bodies, dead bone and tissue are removed from the wound which is then closed to cover the exposed bone. Antibacterial drugs are administered prophylactically till the inflammatory reaction has resolved and the soft tissue wounds have healed satisfactorily. Drainage is provided if suppuration occurs.

Tooth in the line of fracture. In the jaws the fracture line often passes through a tooth socket leaving one side of the root exposed in the wound. The fracture is then compound into the mouth as tearing of the gingival attachment provides a portal of entry to the mouth organisms. Exposed cementum on the surface of the root rapidly dies and repair may not take place between this inert cementum and new bone, so that healing is delayed. As a result of the accident the pulp may become non-vital and a focus of infection. It is wise, therefore, to extract teeth in the line of fracture where there is gross displacement unless they are to be retained temporarily (for ten days) to control a mobile fragment. Where there is little displacement of the fracture the teeth may be kept unless they delay union. The vitality must be checked and non-vital teeth treated as appropriate. In the maxilla vital teeth may be kept, as experience has shown that teeth in the fracture line seldom affect union in the upper jaw.

Reduction of fractures

In reducing fractures the object is to reappose the bone ends as accurately as possible. Although the surgeon should attempt to get perfect reduction the aim is to treat not a radiograph, but a patient, and where displacement is acceptable the patient should not be subjected to unnecessary surgery.

Satisfactory reduction may be impossible where there has been gross comminution or tissue loss, and healing will not take place between the fractured ends if the gap is too wide (over 6 mm). In comminuted fractures all fragments attached to periosteum must be kept.

The best guide to accurate reduction is the occlusion of the teeth, because of the precise way in which the teeth interdigitate. Further, if the occlusion is restored, masticatory function should be satisfactory. In edentulous patients the dentures are the only sound guide. Where they are lost the site of the accident should be searched or a spare set may be available. The fractured jaw is reduced to the sound jaw, but where many teeth are missing or both jaws badly comminuted, the problem is more difficult. The surgeon must then rely more on palpation of the bony margins, the appearance of the patient, and the results shown on post-operative radiographs.

Reduction should be done as soon as possible but where delay is unavoidable it should be remembered that great difficulty will be experienced in reducing maxillary fractures after ten days and mandibular fractures after three weeks.

Immobilisation of the fragments

Any movement in the fracture line after reduction may disturb or tear the granulations or osteoid tissue. It may also cause the bone to heal with a deformity. Some authorities suggest that slight movement in the fracture line may stimulate new bone formation, but the dangers associated with movement heavily outweigh any slight advantage gained. Immobilisation should therefore be complete, and continued till union has taken place, which in the mandible is about four to six weeks and in the maxilla fibrous union is accepted at three to four weeks.

Anaesthesia

Fractures with appreciable displacement are usually reduced under a general anaesthetic. In mandibular fractures a cuffed intranasal endotracheal tube can be passed quite easily but in maxillary fractures involving the nose and ethmoidal bones there is often considerable difficulty, if not danger, in passing a tube through the nose. In these patients the endotracheal tube may be passed through the mouth so that the fractures can be reduced and intraosseous wires or pins put in place. Intermaxillary fixation, however, is completed after the tube has been removed and may present some difficulty. The method of choice for treating these fractures is by traction and where this is not possible the need for a tracheostomy to provide a safe and efficient anaesthetic must be considered.

Where the jaws are to be fixed together under an anaesthetic, a tongue suture is first put through the tongue. This is placed well back to enable the tongue to be drawn forward out of the pharynx. The throat pack is removed and the jaws are then fixed together. Where metal cap splints are used, this can be done with elastics which, in an emergency, are easily cut with scissors. Wires, if used, should be left long for a day so that the twisted ends protrude from the mouth and are easily identified.

Definitive treatment

Soft tissue repair

All wounds are first carefully explored and foreign bodies and dirt removed. Glass is not easy to find and road or coal dust is difficult to get out but if left gives rise to a tattooed scar. To clean wounds or skin abrasions they are gently scrubbed with water, soap and a soft brush, and thoroughly irrigated.

All tissues about the face are precious and, fortunately, because of their rich blood supply, are very viable. Excision is not practised except on tags of loose, dead skin or mucous membrane or round the edges of wounds that are several days old and may have started to epithelialise. Lacerations are then closed in layers by primary suture, with drains inserted where necessary.

Where there has been loss of skin, the edges must not be drawn together under tension as this leads to deformity and scar formation. Full thickness loss in cheek or lips is temporarily repaired by sewing skin to mucous membrane. This prevents scarring, protects the deeper tissues and provides the plastic surgeon with a satisfactory base for his reconstruction.

Tears in the mucosa must be closed to cover exposed bone. Mucous membrane is easier to manipulate than skin so that by undermining edges and rotating flaps deficiencies can usually be made up.

Where bone and soft tissue surgery are being done at the same operation, soft tissue repair is completed after the fractures have been reduced and fixed.

Methods of reduction

Closed reduction – manual. The hands are used to reduce most fresh fractures of both jaws including maxillary fractures of the 'floating' type.

Severe, impacted maxillary fractures may require reduction with forceps (Walsham's or Lion's). One blade of these is placed on the nasal floor and one, covered by rubber tubing, on the palate. The maxilla is drawn downwards and forwards with a strong pull. Rocking may be required to free the bone but this should-be minimal as it can cause damage to other structures.

Closed reduction – traction Traction applies a moderate force continuously over a long period and thereby corrects deformities with little pain or trauma to the patient. It is used for maxillary and mandibular fractures. Intermaxillary traction is applied with arch bars (Fig. 76) or by cementing metal cap splints over the teeth and placing orthodontic elastic bands over the cleats. Where the maxilla is reduced to the mandible this may cause some discomfort if distraction of the temporomandibular joint occurs. Fractures in edentulous patients may be reduced in the same way by using Gunning's splints wired to the jaws.

Open reduction. Mandibular and maxillary fractures may be exposed through an incision in the skin or mucoperiosteum and the bone ends exactly reapposed by direct vision. This method can be used for both jaws and is satisfactory where a wound is present as a result of the accident but, if not, has the disadvantage of leaving a scar. It is often the only way to reduce deformities where treatment has been delayed and malunion has taken place.

Condyles. The fractured condyle head is usually displaced forward and medially by the lateral pterygoid muscle, while the muscles of mastication tend to draw the ascending ramus up and back to produce an anterior open bite, with rotation of the symphysis menti towards the affected side. Reduction is directed to correcting the displacement of the mandible only. This many patients can be taught to do, using their hands at first to assist in re-educating the muscles of mastication. Where swelling and pain make this difficult, and in most bilateral fractures, the mandible is fixed to the maxilla for a week, after which active function is encouraged. In fracture dislocations the same treatment is adequate as it has been shown that, though union occurs in an abnormal position, the head of the condyle remodels to make a functional joint. Where other fractures are present there is no danger of ankylosis if intermaxillary fixation is applied for six weeks.

Reduction of malar bones and zygomatic arch. The external approach devised by Gillies is made through an incision in the skin above the hairline and over the temporal fossa. It is made at an angle to avoid the terminal branches of the superficial temporal artery. The temporal fascia is exposed and incised to give access to an elevator. This is passed deep to the fascia and to the zygomatic arch. It is used to lift the depressed malar forwards, outwards and upwards (Fig. 74). Considerable force is often necessary and the fulcrum must never be the temporal bone, lest the thin lateral wall of the skull be fractured. The assistant's hand is kept on the outer surface of the malar to control its movement and check that reduction is satisfactory. The malar often clicks into place and is stable without fixation but, if not, may be held by an intraosseous pin fixed via a vertical stainless steel rod to a pin in the supraorbital rim or by direct bony wiring at the zygomatic arch, zygomatico-frontal process or the infraorbital rim.

In comminuted fractures the fragments may be reduced via the antrum using a Caldwell–Luc approach. Immobilisation is by direct wiring or by packing the antrum with Whitehead's varnish on ribbon gauze for three weeks.

Fig. 74 Elevation of left malar showing the incision and a lever in place deep to the malar and zygomatic arch. Note the index finger used as a fulcrum to protect the temporal bone.

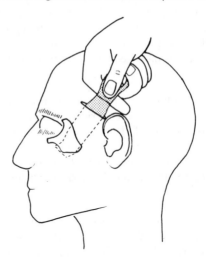

Care must be taken to avoid excessive pressure on the orbital floor lest it damage the contents of the orbit. In multiple maxillary injuries the malar should only be fixed after the rest of the complex has been immobilised. A serious though rare hazard following reduction is bleeding into the floor of the orbit. This may occur during or after operation and results in circumorbital bruising, subconjunctival haemorrhage and proptosis. The pupil is fixed and dilated. Unless the blood is drained from the orbit immediately the sight in the eye may be lost.

Methods of immobilisation

Fractures of the mandible are immobilised by fixing them to the maxilla. A fractured maxilla can be fixed only to the skull and obviously never to the mandible, which is itself a mobile bone. Today many methods of fixation are available but only a few well-tried ones are discussed here. They are of two kinds, those using the teeth or dentures, and intraosseous methods.

Methods using the teeth for fixation

Eyelet wiring. This method is swift, requires no technician or laboratory, and leaves the teeth uncovered so that they can be brought accurately into occlusion. Its disadvantages are that several pairs of sound teeth with a good periodontal condition must be present in each jaw and occlude with similar pairs in the opposite jaw. The eyelet wires are harmless for short periods (six weeks) but in time they tend to loosen the teeth. Finally immobilisation is less satisfactory than with metal cap splints as the wires tend to stretch and loosen.

Eyelets are made by twisting 20 cm lengths of 0.5 mm malleable stainless steel wire (which has first been stretched) round a nail 2 mm in diameter (Fig. 75). Only two turns are made and the tails are cut to equal lengths.

Fig. 75 Eyelet wiring. (*a*) Making eyelet with two twists only of tails. (*b*) Tails of eyelet wire passed between the teeth from buccal side. (*c*) Distal wire passed through the eyelet. (*d*) *Left,* shows correct relationship of wire, flat against the tooth, for twisting. *Right,* incorrect relationship. (*e*) Intermaxillary wire passed from distal aspect of eyelets. (*f*) Intermaxillary wires tightened.

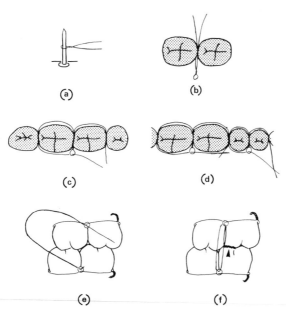

The eyelet is passed from the buccal side between two adjacent teeth below their contact point (Fig. 75b). The tails are then brought round the necks of the teeth below the contact point and out buccally. The posterior tail is passed through the eyelet (Fig. 75c) and the two tails are then firmly twisted up. It is important that the wire is drawn tight round the necks of the teeth below the enamel and the first twist is made as close to the tooth as possible (Fig. 75d). Wires are always twisted clockwise to avoid confusion later when tightening them. Eyelets are put on three or four pairs of teeth as required and on to opposing pairs of teeth in the opposite jaw. Intermaxillary fixation is put in place with a piece of wire passed through corresponding eyelets, and drawn tight and twisted up (Fig. 75e). All wire ends must be turned into the gum or between the teeth to avoid irritating the mucosa.

Arch wiring. This may be suitable where cap splints cannot be constructed or there are inconvenient gaps in the dental arch which make eyelet wiring impossible. A lingual bar, softened by annealing and notched at each edge at 4 mm intervals, is cut into lengths. These are bent to fit closely to the teeth in the upper and lower arches while the fractures are held in their reduced position. Once the arch bar has been tied across the fracture line no further adjustment to the reduction is possible. The bars are lashed to the teeth using 0.5 mm malleable wire. Intermaxillary fixation is put in place round the bars, the notches preventing slipping (Fig. 76).

Cast metal cap splints. These may be used where the patient is not fit enough for a general anaesthetic or where extraoral fixation, usually of the maxilla, is indicated. Their disadvantage is that a laboratory, a technician and time are needed for their construction. Impressions of the jaws are taken with alginate in shallow trays. In severe injuries, pain may make it necessary to premedicate the patient. Where the fragments are displaced separate impressions, each in its own tray, are taken of each segment.

The models are then cast and the surgeon must study the occlusion and the facets on the teeth before articulating the segments. He will then design the splints with the cleats, precision locks, or other special features required and the teeth for extraction marked so that they are left outside the splint. Cleats used for immobilisation are always placed exactly opposite each other on upper and lower splints. The segments of the splints are best not joined at this stage by connecting bars, but localising plates are put on each side of the fractures so that when these have been reduced the locks can be localised and screw connecting bars constructed. Where craniomaxillary fixation is planned two locking plates are necessary to carry the bars to the halo. The procedure for producing the splints in silver alloy is shown in Fig. 77.

The splints are tried in the mouth and adjustments made before they are cemented into place using either cold cure acrylic or black copper cement. Dental wax is run under the cleats and over the locks to protect them from the cement and a solution of sodium bicarbonate is prepared to neutralise

Fig. 76 Arch bar with cleats soldered to it, and with elastic traction in place.

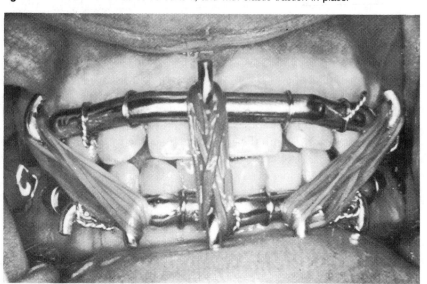

Fig. 77 Cap splint construction. *Above left:* model trimmed down 1 mm round necks of teeth. *Above right:* splint waxed up; wax must be run under the cleats for strength and to eliminate the sharp angle shown on underside of cleat on the left which would prevent easy running of wires. *Below left:* Finished splint back on model, note holes in occlusal surface to allow excess cement to run out and to enable surgeon to check that splint is correctly seated on teeth. *Below right:* Splint with two precision locks and connecting bar crossing the site of fracture.

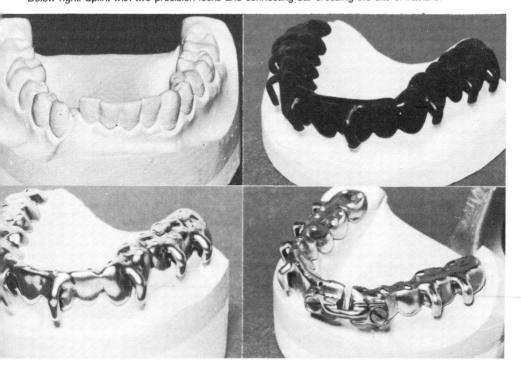

the copper cement if it starts setting before the splint is fitted. The teeth are isolated with cotton wool rolls and dried, using suction and a warm air syringe. The black copper cement is mixed on a cold slab to the consistency of thin cream and poured into the lower splints. These are fitted first to avoid the overspill from the upper falling on the lower teeth. Once in position, all excess cement is removed to prevent inhalation of loose pieces under a general anaesthetic. Traction may be applied after six hours.

When reduction is achieved intermaxillary fixation is effected by binding the cleats with wire. Connecting bars may now be constructed across the fractures and screwed into place (Fig. 78). In the mandible these may provide all the immobilisation necessary so that normal movement can be permitted.

Removal of splints. This is done with orthodontic band removing forceps the occlusal arm of which has been sharpened to penetrate the occlusal surface of the splint. The other beak is carefully inserted under the cervical edge

Fig. 78 (a) The precision lock is in two parts, one plate soldered to the splint and an outer plate which is detachable but is held in position by a screw. (b) Localising wires attached to the outer plates of the precision lock on each side of a fracture are localised with plaster of Paris. (c) A bar is then soldered to the outer plates and screwed across the fracture.

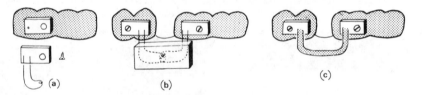

of the splint and by closing the handles the splint is lifted off the teeth (Fig. 79). Care is taken to loosen the appliance (sometimes by dividing it with a dental bur) along its whole length, gradually and equally, to avoid damaging the teeth. The residual cement is removed by scaling.

Craniomaxillary fixation

The maxilla must be fixed to the skull to hold it firmly in place. This is done by attaching metal rods to locking plates on cap splints. These rods come out of the mouth and are connected by means of universal joints (Clouston–Walker joints) and rods to a metal halo frame or intraosseous pins in the supraorbital ridges joined by a connecting bar (Levant frame) (Fig. 80).

Halo head frame. This is screwed to the head by means of pins which penetrate the skin and engage the outer bony cortical plate of the skull. Two pairs of opposing pins in the occipital and frontal regions are placed above the hairline to avoid unsightly scars. The temporal vessels should be identified to avoid damage to these when placing the frontal pins. Once in position rods from metal cap splints on the teeth will provide rigid fixation of the maxilla (Fig. 81).

Supraorbital pins and frame. Metal pins inserted into the lateral part of the supraorbital ridges are connected by a Levant frame. To place the pins an incision is made in the eyebrow and holes drilled into the supraorbital bone using a brace and bit. A self-tapping pin is inserted to engage both cortical plates without penetrating the inner. The pins are then joined using a Levant frame and this connected to the teeth via rods. The advantage of this system is greater comfort for the patient. (Fig. 80).

Fig. 79 Removal of cap splints using modified orthodontic band removing forceps. One sharp beak pierces the occlusal surface of the splint whilst the other beak lifts the cervical edge of the splint.

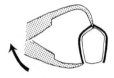

Fig. 80 Levant frame attached to upper metal cap splint by bars and universal joints. Note facial laceration extended for open reduction.

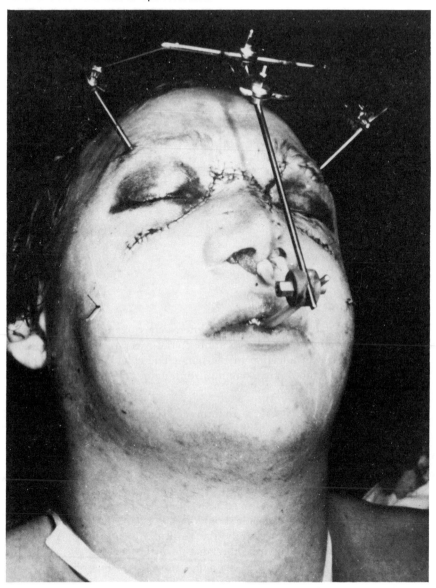

Internal suspension. In Le Fort I fractures 0.5 stainless steel wire is passed round the zygomatic arches using an awl inserted through the mucosa beneath the arch in the upper buccal sulcus. A wire is threaded through the hole in the awl and drawn upwards over the zygomatic arch and back down on the lateral side into the mouth. This wire is attached either to cleats on metal cap splints or eyelet wires (Fig. 82).

Fig. 81 *Left:* Royal Berkshire halo. Note screw for fixation to the outer cortical table of cranium. *Right:* Gunning's splints mounted on occlusion. Note hole anteriorly for feeding.

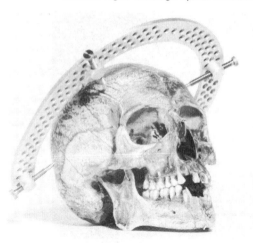 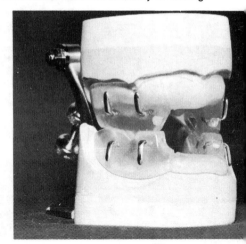

Interosseous methods of fixation

The excellent apposition provided by interosseous fixation results in rapid healing and, if inserted under an antibacterial cover and sterile conditions, rarely gives rise to infection in the bone. The chief contraindications in interosseous methods are comminuted fractures and those which are infected at presentation.

Interosseous wiring of the mandible. All forms described here will rapidly become loose unless supported by effective intermaxillary fixation. The upper border is used where a tooth in line has been extracted or where the fracture is compound into the mouth. Buccal and lingual flaps are made to expose both sides of the fracture line. Holes are drilled through the bone. They are placed deep to the reflection of the mucosa to bury the wire more effectively, and at least 5 m from the alveolar crest, but avoiding the inferior dental nerve. The anterior hole should be lower than that on the posterior fragment to overcorrect slightly the vertical displacement. A 0.5 mm malleable stainless steel wire is threaded through the holes, twisted up, the ends cut short, turned in, and the flap sutured back (Fig. 83).

Wiring at the lower border of the mandible is indicated in compound injuries through the skin where the bone is already exposed and in those fractures where upper border wiring is not possible. Two centimeters below the lower border an incision is made which may follow the curve of the jaw at the angle, but must be kept 2.5 cm below the lobe of the ear to avoid the facial nerve. The bone is exposed and, with a periosteal elevator is cleaned of muscle attachment both buccally and lingually for 2 cm above the lower margin. The fracture line is identified and one fragment is grasped with a

Fig. 82 Internal suspension of fractured maxilla. *Left:* wire around zygomatic arch; *Right:* wire suspended from wire at zygomatico-frontal suture.

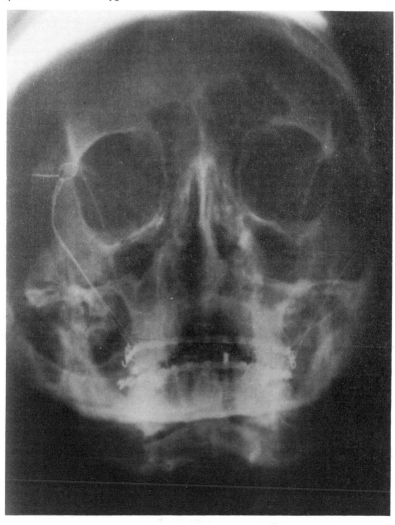

pair of bone-holding forceps. These have a hole which admits the bur whilst protecting the lingual soft tissues. Holes are drilled on the two fragments so that when the fracture is reduced the line joining them is at 90° to the fracture line. They must also be cut parallel to the buccolingual direction of the fracture to ensure that they open on to the lingual cortical plate. The lower hole should be 0.5 cm above the lower border. When prepared in this way a wire passed through the holes and twisted up will control the displacement. Greater security will be achieved by threading the wire to make a figure eight which crosses over at the lower border (Fig. 83).

Fig. 83 (a) Upper border wiring by simple wire ligature through the outer plate of a tooth socket. (b) Lower border figure-of-eight wiring. (c) Lower border simple wire ligature. Upward displacement of the posterior fragment (shown by dotted lines) may occur if the ligature is incorrectly placed. Anterior ligature shows correct positioning of the holes and ligature.

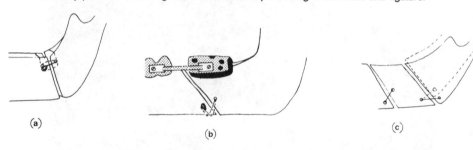

(a)

(b)

(c)

Interosseus wiring in maxillary fractures. This is a very satisfactory method of fixation where the bony buttresses can be used, but is not suitable for thin plates of bone.

Plating. Plating of the mandible has the advantage that intermaxillary fixation is only necessary whilst the plate is being placed. Small malleable plates of titanium or stainless steel are inserted across the fracture line via an intraoral approach. The incision is made through the mucoperiosteum below the attached gingivae. The fracture line is identified and the plate adapted to the contour of the bone. Holes are drilled in the outer cortical bone for two screws on each side of the fracture. In the anterior region of the mandible two plates are placed across the fracture line to counteract the increased torsional forces (Fig. 84). Compression plates are popular with some surgeons. They are placed at the lower border of the mandible to compress the fractured ends together when the screws are tightened. Removal of plates once healing has occurred is considered necessary for compression plates while opinions vary on malleable plates. Where the metal becomes exposed or infection supervenes, plates must be removed.

Intraosseous pins. These are seldom used now but have an application in comminuted or infected fractures because they can be inserted at a distance from the fracture line. They may be used in malar fractures to fix these to a head frame.

The edentulous posterior fragment of the mandible

The edentulous posterior fragment may consist of only a part of the ascending ramus or may include a considerable part of the body. It is controlled in various ways.

Impaction against the body. Where the fracture is both vertically and horizontally favourable the posterior fragment may be held in place by the body when this is immobilised. Where displacement might take place this may be acceptable because movement is limited by the periosteum.

Fig. 84 *Upper:* Radiograph shows plating of mandibular fractures. *Lower:* Use of miniplates in the middle third of the face.

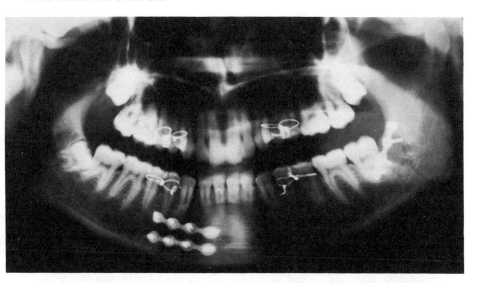

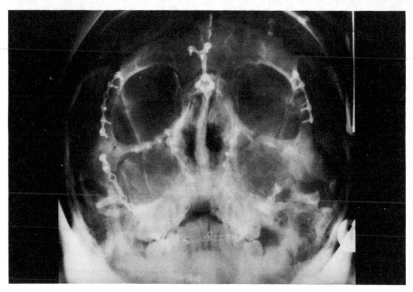

Tooth in line. Where the only tooth on the posterior fragment is a molar in the line of fracture, the extraction of which will render the posterior fragment edentulous, this may be retained temporarily. The removal of its anterior root from the fracture line by amputation and thereby leaving interradicular bone, and not cementum, exposed in the lesion has been successfully used.

Interosseous fixation. Plating of the fracture is the most satisfactory method of fixation. Where this system is not available upper or lower border wiring with intermaxillary fixation is used.

Edentulous jaws

Though edentulous jaws should be reduced and fixed to obtain satisfactory union, in many cases displacement will be prevented by the periosteum and slight deformity can be compensated by construction of new dentures. Open reduction which involves stripping of the periosteum must be avoided.

Dentures. The patient's dentures may be used as a splint after removing the anterior teeth to make a space for feeding. These are often immediately available and have the advantage of reproducing both the alveolar ridge and the patient's bite accurately. As they have no cleats, holes are bored through them to pass wires for intermaxillary fixation. Where there is no displacement the dentures may be worn wired together and the jaws immobilised by a firm bandage.

Gunning's splints. These are the standard splint for immobilising edentulous jaws. They are an upper and lower bite block made in acrylic. They have a shallow periphery, a hole anteriorly for feeding, and cleats and precision locks for intermaxillary fixation. They are constructed from casts of the patient's dentures, which are also used to register the bite, or by direct impressions of the patient's jaws when the bite is registered using conventional bite blocks (Fig. 81).

Where there is displacement neither a satisfactory impression nor bite recording is possible, and the fitting surface of the splint is lined with gutta-percha and moulded to the jaw *after* the fragments have been reduced. By placing gutta-percha in previously prepared gutters on the occlusal surface, the bite can also be corrected before putting intermaxillary fixation in place.

These splints may be wired together and the jaws kept immobilised with a bandage, but this is not satisfactory, except for the simplest fracture.

Circumferential and transalveolar wiring. Gunning's splints or dentures may be wired to the jaws to hold the bone fragments firmly in place. Suitable grooves are cut in the occlusal, buccal and lingual surface of the splints to accommodate the wires.

In the lower jaw three wires are used, one on each side in the first molar region and one anteriorly. The wire is put in place by passing a curved Kelsey Fry awl (Fig. 85a) through the mucuous membrane at the lingual reflection whilst the denture is kept in place to localise the position of the wires. The awl is passed down to, and through, the skin at the lower border, keeping the point as close to bone as possible to avoid the lingual and facial arteries. A 0.5 mm malleable stainless steel wire is passed through the eye (Fig 85a) and drawn up into the mouth. The wire is detached and clipped

Fig. 85 Circumferential wiring. (a) Kelsey Fry awl passed lingual to the mandible. (b) Wire alongside lingual side of mandible and the awl passed bucally to pick up extraoral end of the wire. (c) Sawing through soft tissue to ensure close apposition of wire on bone. (d) Lower splint lined with gutta-percha wired in place. (e) *Left*, straight awl passed through maxillary alveolus and across the antral floor to draw transalveolar wire through from palate. *Right*, transalveolar wire in place to hold upper Gunning's splint.

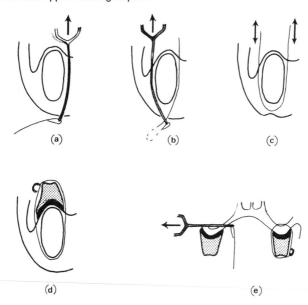

with artery forceps at both ends. The awl is then passed buccally and brought out through the same skin incision. The wire is then threaded through the awl and drawn up on the buccal side (Fig. 84b). A sawing movement is used to cut through the soft tissues over the lower border as the wire must rest closely against bone, lest it become loose during treatment. When all three wires are in place they are drawn tight round the lower splint and twisted up (Fig. 84d). An alternative method is to pass the wires through an extraoral stab incision up into the mouth.

The upper splint, which should have no palate, is held in position by transalveolar wires, one on each side in the molar region and one anteriorly. With the splint in the mouth, a straight Kelsey Fry awl is passed from the buccal side above the periphery through the alveolus to emerge on the palate. The lateral wires should pass over the antral floor as its cortical plate then prevents them cutting through. Great care is taken not to twist the awl lest the point break off in bone. A wire is now threaded through the eye of the awl and drawn back through the bone. Once all three wires are in place they are twisted up to tie the splint in place (Fig. 85e).

Intermaxillary fixation or craniomaxillary fixation may be used by putting locking plates on the Gunning splints to carry bars to a head frame.

After-care

After-care must include special attention to oral hygiene and diet, which have been discussed in Chapter II. In addition the patient may require antibacterial drugs to be administered prophylactically for a period, particularly in comminuted or compound fractures and where intraosseus wiring or pins have been used for immobilisation.

Those patients who have minor fractures, who have satisfactory healing of skin or mucous membrane, and who have no extraoral forms of fixation may continue treatment as out-patients. Those who do not have their lower jaw immobilised may be allowed to work if they have a desk job. The necessity for regular oral hygiene must be stressed.

Follow-up examination of the fracture. The patient must be reviewed at regular intervals to check that the splints and intermaxillary fixation are firm and in their correct position. Wounds must be regularly examined and where plates are used, checked for exposure of the metal. Examination for union is done by removing the intermaxillary fixation or connecting bars between splints and testing for mobility.

Radiographs. These should be taken immediately after reduction and fixation to ensure that the position is satisfactory. They may be repeated during treatment whenever it is suspected that displacement has occured in the fracture, or where there are signs of infection.

The fracture in the mandible will not show signs of callus formation for several months, that is, long after clinical union should have taken place. The fracture line may show on radiographs anything up to a year after the accident that is, till cortical bone has re-formed.

Removal of splints. This is done as soon as clinical union occurs. No anaesthetic is necessary, even for removal of circumferential and transalveolar wires or pins. Interosseus wires, if symptomless, are left in place indefinitely but the patient must be told of their presence.

Rehabilitation. Treatment is not complete till dead and loose teeth still present have been treated by root filling or extraction, missing teeth replaced with dentures or bridges, and full masticatory function restored.

Complications of fractures

Delayed union

Normally fractures unite in about four to eight weeks, but take longer in elderly patients. This time may be greatly increased in comminuted, compound or infected fractures. Some may take several months to heal, during which time they must be kept immobilised. Radiographs should be taken at intervals to determine whether smoothing of the bone ends and eburnation, indicating non-union, has occurred.

Malunion

This is union with the bone ends still misplaced or badly reduced. It may be slight and cause the patient little disability or it may be such as to interfere with function or appearance. Slight deformity affecting the occlusion can be treated by grinding or extracting teeth, and the provision of dentures. More severe deformities may require re-fracture and re-apposition of the bone ends by an open operation. Once the decision has been made to correct the defect surgically the operation should not be long delayed.

Non-union

This term refers to the failure to obtain bony union, where healing has occurred by fibrous union only. In facial trauma it is of significance only in the mandible. Clinically movement is found across the fracture line. On radiographs a smoothing over of the bone ends is seen, which is later followed by a deposition of cortical bone (eburnation). The chief causes of non-union are a failure to achieve satisfactory apposition, bone loss, and movement or infection in the fracture line.

Bone loss. In severe injuries, particularly in gunshot wounds, there may be bone loss. In the mandible, if this is slight, a satisfactory result can be achieved by approximating the bone ends. Otherwise, the gap is accepted and the fragments are reduced into their normal position and held there by splints, long bone plates or external pin fixation. When soft tissue healing has taken place and the inflammatory reaction has settled the defect is repaired with bone grafts. This may be delayed several weeks, or even months.

Movement. This can tear or damage the granulations or young osteoid tissue concerned in repair. Shearing movement, that is vertical movement of the bone ends parallel to the line of fracture, is more damaging than a bending movement which tends to leave the majority of the granulations intact at the centre of the axis.

Infection. This may reach the fracture from wounds in the skin or more commonly from the mouth.

The mandible is more susceptible to infection than the maxilla. In the latter drainage is downward into the mouth and the thin plates of bone with a good blood supply make it more resistant to infection.

Infection from the mouth may enter the fracture through a tear in the mucous membrane, from dead teeth, particularly those in the line of fracture, or by direct or lymphatic spread from other infected teeth in the jaw. At an early stage radiographs show a resorption of the bone ends and widening of the fracture line. Energetic treatment with antibacterial drugs and drainage is necessary lest the infection progress to an osteomyelitis.

Treatment. Treatment of non-union is necessary in the body of the mandible but may be acceptable in the ascending ramus and the condyle, if function is satisfactory. Treatment is by open reduction, freshening of the bone ends and interosseous wiring, or bone grafting if necessary.

Residual trismus

This may be caused by bony interference which occurs when the zygoma has been badly reduced and the coronoid process impacts against the displaced zygomatic arch. It may result from extrinsic scars or rarely from fibrous ankylosis in the temporomandibular joint following intracapsular fractures of the condyle. The cause must always be carefully sought and corrected either surgically or by the use of exercises and physiotherapy.

Further reading

Killey, H. C. (1981), *Fractures of the Middle Third of the Facial Skeleton*, 4th edn. John Wright, Bristol.

Killey, H. C. (1983), *Fractures of the Mandible*, 3rd edn. John Wright, Bristol.

Rowe, N. L. and Williams, J. L., eds. (1985). *Maxillofacial Injuries*. Churchill Livingstone, Edinburgh.

xv Considerations in the treatment of tumours of the mouth

Tumours of the mouth are classified according to the cells from which they originate. *It is outside the scope of this book to discuss the histology, signs and symptoms of each type of tumour.* In treatment it is the nature of the tumour which is important, that is, whether the growth is benign, locally invasive or malignant.

Benign tumours. These are slow-growing and encapsulated. Histologically the cells and the stroma are well differentiated. Their symptoms are swelling and, occasionally, the results of pressure on adjacent structures. In the mouth papilloma, fibroma, fibrous epulis, lipoma, osteoma, chrondroma and the odontomes are benign tumours. When removed they do not recur.

Locally invasive tumours. These have most of the characteristics of benign tumours except that they infiltrate into the surrounding tissue. As a result they cannot be satisfactorily enucleated or curetted out and, unless a wide excision is made, they may recur locally. On the other hand, they do not usually form metastases either in the lymph nodes or in other parts of the body. Locally invasive tumours in the mouth are giant cell reparative granuloma, osteoclastoma, myxoma, adenoma, and pleomorphic adenoma.

Malignant tumours. These are of rapid growth and are not encapsulated. Histologically the cells present as well or poorly differentiated, and the stroma is very scanty. When they reach the skin or mucosa they ulcerate through to produce a fungating ulcer. They metastasise by infiltrating the lymphatics or capillaries, by forming emboli and by transplanation to start tumours in other parts of the body. In the mouth squamous cell carcinoma, sarcoma, multiple myeloma, adenocarcinoma and melanoma are all found, squamous cell carcinoma being the commonest. The study of malignant tumours is called oncology.

Hamartomas. These developmental abnormalities are not true tumours but have some similar features. Those found in the mouth are haemangiomas and lymphomangiomas.

Diagnosis and assessment.

Oral cancer is often asymptomatic in the early stages and late presentation is not uncommon. Prognosis can be improved by early detection and the dental surgeon has an important role in the early diagnosis as the more common tumours are usually easily seen on careful examination. Malignant lesions of lip, tongue and floor of mouth have a comparatively high rate of cure if treatment is started when the growth is small.

History

The most important points are the age of the patient, as certain tumours occur in particular age groups, and the rate of growth of the tumour. Symptoms involving adjacent nerves are important as paraesthesia or paralysis may be caused by their involvement in malignant tumours and is rarely a symptom of pressure from a benign growth. Pain is a late symptom in malignant tumours. Smoking and drinking habits are of interest as chronic irritation of the oral mucosa by alcohol or smoking may cause leukoplakia which is considered a precancerous condition.

Examination

Care is taken to look at all accessible parts of the mouth especially the undersurface of the tongue, pillars of the fauces and the posterior part of the tongue and palate. The examination is directed to establishing the site, size and shape of the lesion. The edges of the swelling are well defined in benign tumours but may merge into the host tissues in invasive neoplasms. It is important to ascertain whether the swelling is fixed to the overlying skin or mucosa or to the underlying bone or muscle. The consistency, colour and the presence of ulceration are noted. Malignant ulcers typically have everted edges with a necrotic base and are surrounded by an area of granulation tissue often indurated owing to the host's attempt to wall off the tumour. Unlike traumatic ulcers, they fail to heal spontaneously after the local irritation, such as sharp teeth or ill-fitting dentures, has been removed.

The lymph nodes draining the area should be palpated. In early malignancy the nodes are palpable, often being very hard and non-tender. Later they become fixed to adjacent tissues when the tumour breaks through the capsule of the node. Where ulceration of the growth has occurred with subsequent superimposed infection the secondary malignant nodes may become enlarged and tender.

Radiography

Tumours in bone require radiographs in two planes to show their extent. To demonstrate fine changes in the bone it is necessary to take films at different exposures. Benign soft tissue tumours such as fibromas and neuromas show as rounded radiolucent areas very like a dental cyst except that there is no well-defined cortical plate. Calcified benign tumours such as central osteoma or odontomes are separated from normal bone by a radiolucent line representing the capsule round the lesion.

Of the locally invasive tumours, the ameloblastoma occurs chiefly in the mandible and is of two types: the monocystic which on radiographs looks very like a dental cyst, except that its margins have a lobulated outline and the multicystic, which has a multiloculated appearance with well-differentiated trabeculae and a scalloped margin. Adjacent tooth roots are displaced or often resorbed. The central giant cell reparative granuloma

Fig. 86 Radiographs of malignant tumours of jaws. *Above:* Carcinoma of maxillary antrum invading extraction socket. Note destruction of bone. *Below:* Carcinoma of mandible showing extensive diffuse bone destruction.

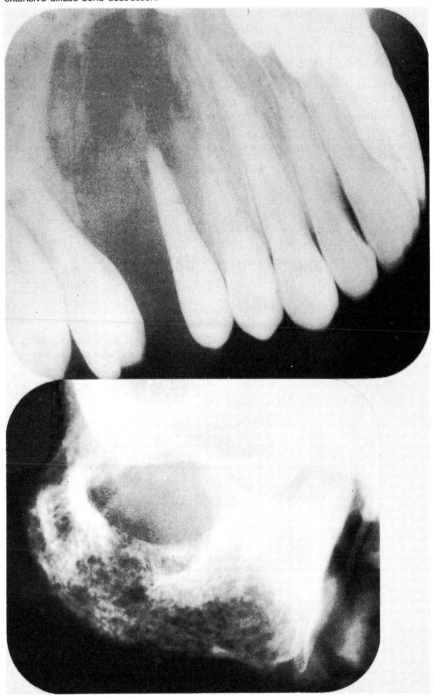

also has a multilocular appearance and adjacent tooth roots too are often resorbed. Where this tumour is suspected the blood chemistry should be investigated and the hands, pelvis, and long bones radiographed for other lesions lest the patient be suffering from some general disease such as hyperparathyroidism. It is important but difficult to diagnose a central haemangioma from radiographs. It is said to present as indefinite areas of resorption which give a soap-bubble effect.

Primary or secondary carcinoma in bone has an appearance similar to that of osteomyelitis except that no sequestra are seen and the patient has no inflammatory symptoms. Sarcoma may either be osteolytic, with gross bone destruction, or osteoplastic, when bone destruction and irregular new bone formation, sometimes with a sun-ray appearance, are seen in the same film.

Computerised tomography (C.T. Scanning) is now routinely used in diagnosis and treatment planning for tumours, particularly those in soft tissues. In this technique the area under investigation is scanned by an X-ray beam in multiple planes sequentially. A computer calculates the absorption of the X-rays and a picture of a horizontal section of the body is produced (Fig. 87).

Magnetic resonance imaging (M.R.I.) is a relatively new technique which has the advantage of producing an image with great tissue contrast without using ionising radiation. The extent of tumours can be visualised well with this technique.

The uptake of radioactive isotopes (e.g. iodine, technetium) by tissues can be used in their investigation (radioscintiscan). Following an intravenous injection of the isotope the area is scanned with a gamma camera. The differential uptake of the isotope between the normal tissue and a tumour may give an indication of its extent.

Aspiration

It is wise to attempt aspiration of all well circumscribed radiolucent central tumours before excision to eliminate the possibility of their being cysts or central haemanigomas (see page 163).

Biopsy

The true nature of a new growth can only be established by histological examination. This will show the capsule if it is present and the nature of the cells and the nature of the stroma forming the tumour. Its activity can be assessed by interpreting the degrees of dysplasia present in tissue sections. To obtain a specimen for histological examination all or part of the tumour may be excised. Although a diagnostic biopsy is essential a more cautious attitude is prevalent today towards removing portions of suspected malignant tumours too long before operation because this can cause spread through the lymphatics and blood vessels.

Fig. 87 Computerised tomography. *Upper,* lateral view showing lines of cuts for scan. *Below,* C.T. scan showing tumour of antrum: note extension into nasal cavity and through lateral bony wall.

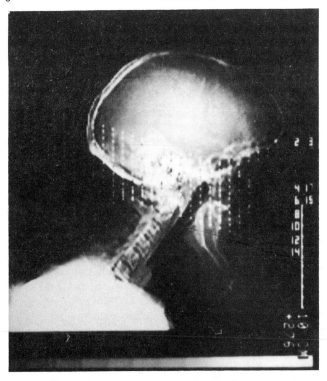

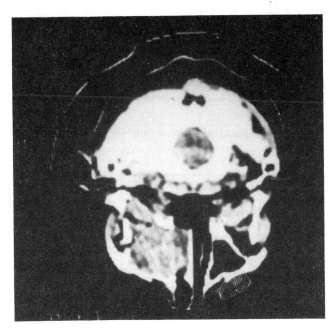

Excisional biopsy. In this the whole of the tumour is excised at one operation, and is sent for biopsy. This procedure requires a diagnosis of new growth to be made from the history, the clinical examination and the radiographs. It is indicated for all tumours which are obviously benign and for those locally invasive or malignant tumours where the diagnosis is beyond reasonable doubt and the radical operation required is not disfiguring or incapacitating.

Incisional biopsy. Removal of part of the tumour is used for locally invasive or malignant tumours where the diagnosis is in doubt, or where a major operation of a disfiguring nature is necessary to eradicate the growth. It is also taken where assessment of the rate of growth or degree of differentiation of the tumour cells is important in deciding the form (surgery or radiotherapy) that treatment should take.

A satisfactory specimen is excised of sufficient size to enable a representative histological section of the tumour to be prepared. It must include a margin of normal tissue, particularly the junction between this and the growth and also the superficial tissues covering the tumour. Ulcerated areas are of little value as the necrotic tissue and local inflammatory response may mask the nature of the lesion. A wedge or ellipse is cut out with a knife and not electrosurgery, which may 'fry' the specimen and make it useless for diagnostic purposes. It is fixed at once by placing in ten per cent formalin in physiological saline and sent to the laboratory with a full history and description of the lesion.

As this minor procedure may cause spread of malignant tumours it is generally agreed that partial biopsies should be performed immediately before treatment with surgery or radiotherapy is commenced by a surgeon who is prepared to complete any major surgical procedures necessary. In this respect frozen sections give a very quick result but are unfortunately considered somewhat unreliable.

A diagnosis may also be made on material obtained by fine needle aspiration (lymph nodes) or by punch biopsy where a core of tissue is removed. A hollow drill in a dental engine will remove a core from a central bone tumour. Smears of mucosal lesions (cytology) may be collected, and the results rely on sampling technique and assessment by an experienced cytopathologist.

Treatment of tumours

At present surgery is the only safe and satisfactory treatment for benign and locally invasive tumours. Cryosurgery, destroying tissue by freezing at low temperatures, has an increasing application, as does the use of laser surgery. This technique produces vaporisation of the tissue, allowing precise excision of dysplastic lesions. Both techniques are relatively pain-free post-operatively, with the minimum amount of wound contraction.

Fig. 88 Excision of pedunculated tumour. (*a*) Lifting tumour gently to incise round its base. (*b*) Tumour lifted so that base can be cut through at a greater depth.

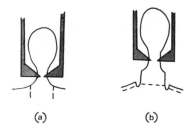

(a)   (b)

Benign tumours

Excision of pedunculated tumours.   Papilloma, fibroma, fibrous epulis and (rarely) lipoma may be pedunculated. The tumour is grasped with toothed forceps and an incision is made round its base through the whole depth of the mucosa and submucosa, with a wide margin to ensure its entire removal. It is then drawn up out of the tissues and the base cut free. The edges of the wound are undermined to facilitate closure without tension. Tumours arising from the mucoperiosteum are excised in the same way except that the periosteum is removed with the base (Fig. 88).

Sessile tumours.   These are removed through an incision in the mucous membrane, care being taken not to incise the tumour. It is shelled out easily by blunt dissection. Haemostasis is important as a large haematoma may form in the cavity (Fig. 89).

Tumours in the hard palate.   These may be completely excised with the overlying mucoperiosteum. The deficiency is then covered with a Whitehead's varnish dressing sutured into place to cover the raw bone which granulates rapidly.

Osteoma.   Superficial osteomas may be excised with chisels or burs. Osteomas and odontomes in bone may be removed in the same way as a buried tooth or root (Chapter VIII).

Locally invasive tumours

Tumours on the gingiva.   The tumour commonly found is a giant cell reparative granuloma. This presents as an epulis, usually in the premolar or anterior region of the mouth. It should be excised with a wide margin of at least 0.5 cm of normal gum tissue and the underlying periosteum removed with the tumour, together with the underlying cortical bone. Frequently the tumour extends between the teeth to involve the lingual aspect of the gingivae. To avoid a recurrence the teeth involved should be extracted, the interdental papilla and lingual mucosa excised and the underlying bone removed to the depth of a few millimetres. The raw area is then covered with a pack held in place with sutures.

Fig. 89 Excision of sessile tumour; lipoma of floor of mouth.

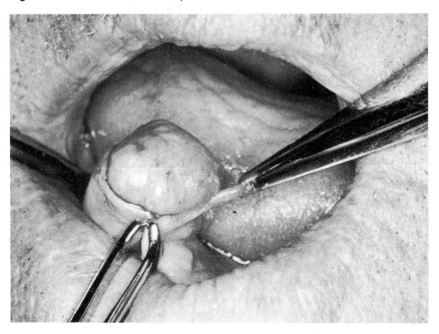

Soft tissue tumours. These include pleomorphic adenoma in the cheek, palate and lip, and lymphangioma and haemangioma in the cheek, lip and tongue.

The pleomorphic adenoma is usually encapsulated but is very friable and may tear so that portions are retained. It is widely excised to ensure total removal.

Haemangiomas and lymphangiomas are usually congenital and grow chiefly during the early years of life. Angiography and computerised tomography are important in diagnosis and treatment planning for haemangiomas. They are best left untreated unless they give rise to symptoms such as haemorrhage, or are increasing markedly in size. Larger lesions require embolisation and selective vessel ligation. Excision with a clear margin of sound tissue is suitable for smaller lesions. Blood should be available for transfusion and the main vessels to the part may need to be tied off to control bleeding. Haemangiomas can be dissected out with diathermy, which does control haemorrhage but leaves an ugly wound, or treated with cryosurgery.

The extraction of teeth near a haemangioma may be followed by excessive bleeding if the tumour is torn and every effort should be made pre-operatively for the adequate control of haemorrhage.

Central bone tumours. These include amelobastoma, central giant cell reparative granuloma and haemangioma. Locally invasive tumours in bone are sometimes difficult to differentiate from benign central tumours or even cysts, and are often so large that their complete removal with a satisfactory margin is a mutilating operation that may affect both the patient's function and his appearance. As these tumours do not metastasise, the final diagnosis is made by taking a specimen for biopsy before operation. Where a central haemangioma is suspected, specimens cannot be taken without special preparation as bleeding may be so extensive that massive transfusion and ligature of both carotid arteries are necessary as life-saving measures.

In the mandible, operations on locally invasive tumours are planned, if possible, to leave sufficient bone at the lower border to maintain the continuity of the jaw. Before operation metal cap splints are prepared. At operation the mandible is exposed, intraorally, if the continuity of the lower border is to be maintained, and the tumour is excised with a margin of half to one centimetre of normal bone on all sides. The inferior dental alveolar nerve is preserved wherever possible. Intermaxillary fixation is put in place to support the jaw.

Where the continuity of the mandible cannot be maintained, metal cap splints are fitted as before and the jaw exposed from the lower border. The bone is stripped of periosteum and healthy mucoperiosteum, but the mucosa involved by the tumour is removed. The tumour, with a clear margin of normal bone, is cut out with burs, chisels or a Gigli saw. Where continuity of the oral mucosa has been maintained a graft taken from a rib or from the iliac crest is suitably tailored, fixed into place using wires or malleable plates and packed round with bone chips at the same operation, otherwise this is delayed until mucosal healing has taken place. The jaw is immobilised with splints or with pin fixation until the graft takes.

Maxillary tumours are excised widely, usually through an intraoral approach. Splints are required to carry an obturator to place in the deficiency caused by removal of large tumours, or may hold skin grafts or dressings in place over large raw areas. Initially the obturator is secured in place using internal fixation such as transpalatal wires.

Malignant tumours

The treatment of malignant tumours is planned jointly by a team consisting of a surgeon, radiotherapist and chemotherapist. The latter has, at present, little place in the treatment of malignancy occurring in the head and neck with the exception of generalised diseases such as the lymphomas. Generally surgery is the treatment of choice for tumours of bones and radiotherapy is used successfully on sensitive growths of the soft tissues. In many cases to achieve the best possible result both are used in the same patient. Surgery may precede or follow radiotherapy. Where it is done first the risk of radionecrosis is reduced if wound healing is complete before the area is irradiated. When surgery follows radiotherapy difficulty in healing may occur owing to the reduced blood supply as a result of the local endarteritis. In a combined treatment surgery may be used to remove the main tumour mass and radiotherapy is directed to the more inaccessible remaining tissue and lymphatic fields, hopefully as a cure, but more often as a means of palliation.

Fig. 90 Radiograph shows ameloblastoma of mandible; *note* multiocular appearance.

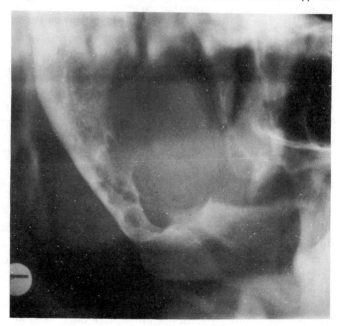

Surgery

Surgery of malignant tumours is planned to cover three aspects. First, the total removal of the tumour, together with a very wide margin of apparently normal tissue. Second, if the lymphatic system is involved the excision of the lymphatic vessels draining the area with all the nodes involved is required. In tumours of the mouth this includes the submandibular, and upper and lower deep cervical nodes. The operation aims to remove all lymphatic, connective and muscular tissue in the area of drainage in one block, which in the neck is limited above by the mylohyoid muscle, anteriorly by the midline of the neck, posteriorly by the trapezius muscle and below by the clavicle. The structures removed include not only the lymphatics but also the submandibular and sometimes the parotid salivary glands and the sternomastoid and mylohyoid muscles. Finally, the area must be repaired.

Adequate access is important for successful tumour excision and this may require splitting the upper or lower lip. The mandible can be sectioned and repositioned with wires or plates at the end of surgery.

At operation the first consideration is to cover the raw areas either by primary closure of the mucosa, by suturing mucous membrane to skin or by grafts. Where bone has been removed from the mandible and immediate grafting is not performed, prevention of contraction causing displacement of the fragments is important so that later reconstructive surgery becomes difficult.

Fig. 91 Carcinoma of alveolus showing typical fungating appearance with sloughing.

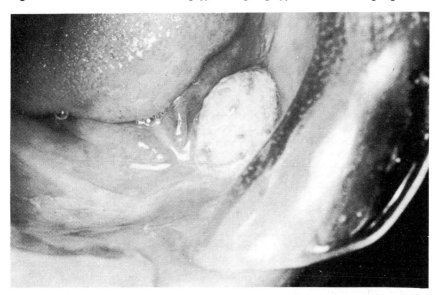

A metal or an acrylic implant or external pin fixation may be used to maintain the bone ends in their correct relationship. Nowadays reconstructive surgery is usually performed at the initial operation. This may include bone grafting and the use of different flap procedures to cover the soft tissue defect. The advent of microvascular surgery has introduced the vascularised flap to oral reconstructive surgery. An example is the use of the radial forearm flap (including skin, muscle and bone) whose dependent arteries and veins are connected to vessels in the neck, providing a viable flap which is both functional and aesthetically acceptable. In some instances it may be necessary to provide some form of cosmetic or functional prosthesis to help the patient's rehabilitation.

Radiotherapy

Biological effects of radiation. X-ray, gamma ray and, less commonly, high-energy electron or neutron beams produced by suitable machines are used in the treatment of malignant tumours. Alternatively, radioactive materials can be inserted into the tissues around the lesion or placed into a mould designed to fit the area to be irradiated. As the ionising radiations pass through the tissues they are absorbed and remove electrons from atoms thus altering the cell molecules which leads to chemical changes. These in turn result in biological effects including lethal damage to living cells. Such effects are more pronounced in tissues whose cells are undergoing frequent division. Modern megavoltage X-rays are capable of much greater penetration in tissue than the older lower-voltage forms.

Considerations in the treatment of tumours of the mouth   **215**

The effectiveness of radiotheraphy depends on the sensitivity of the malignant cells and the effect on the normal surrounding tissues. Treatment is usually in repeated doses until the total planned dose is given, daily over a period of 4–6 weeks.

Radiation therapy produces damage to the normal tissues which usually proliferate and recover. The tumour regresses and is replaced by scar tissue. The mucosa becomes inflamed and hypersensitive but recovers within 12 weeks after completion of therapy. Irradiation of the salivary glands results in reduced, thickened saliva. The patient develops a dry mouth and their sense of taste is lost. Dryness of the mouth contributes to the discomfort experienced in chewing and swallowing, for which local anaesthetic lozenges or Benzydamine hydrochloride mouthwash may be prescribed. A high standard of oral hygiene must be maintained, including rinsing after all meals with bland mouthwashes (1 per cent Chlorhexidine). Foods should be soft, easily masticated and of high nutritional content.

Effects of radiation on bone. All tissues that have received a cancercidal dose of radiation develop an endarteritis. In bone the periosteum becomes thickened and avascular; osteoblasts and osteoclasts are absent, so that rapair after injury is slow or does not take place. In children, bone growth is retarded and the dentition is abnormal. Radiation osteomyelitis occurs in the mandible sometimes years after the treatment and is always secondary to a latent necrosis. It appears after minor injury, especially where there is a breach in the alveolar mucosa, particularly after tooth extraction. Radiographically the earliest changes are a 'moth-eaten' appearance of the bone, followed by sequestration often involving the whole bone from the angle to the canine region. Most cases present in a subacute manner with a painful, indurated swelling of the lower jaw, and slight pyrexia. The diagnosis is made from the history and the radiographic appearance.

Treatment is conservative. A high standard of general nutrition and, during the sub-acute phase, a course of antibiotics for two to four weeks, may prevent sequestration. Local treatment is confined to irrigation and removal of the sequestra when they separate. The results of natural healing may be quite satisfactory although the process is somewhat drawn out. Pain varies in intensity, and where simple analgesics fail relief may be obtained by giving an inferior dental injection with 1–2 ml of 95 per cent alcohol or performing a trigeminal root section.

Pre-radiation dental care. The radiotherapist will invite the assistance of the dental surgeon for several reasons. Death of bone may follow irradiation and the extraction of teeth or severe periodontal disease may start a radiation osteomyelitis. The mucosal reaction is always severe in septic tissues and is increased by metal fillings which give rise to a heavy election emission when irradiated. Reactions of the mucosa may mean limiting radiation and underdosage of the tumour. Poor oral hygiene and lack of saliva due to fibrosis of the salivary glands commonly causes rampant caries and advanced periodontal disease of similar distribution to that seen in the mouths of those who have xerostomia for other reasons. Further, because of impairment of the blood supply of the jaws, there is the added danger that extraction of the teeth may be followed by infected sockets and osteomyelitis, particularly of the mandible.

In an attempt to avoid these sequelae it was common practice to remove all teeth before such treatment started. Unfortunately this does not always prevent osteoradionecrosis, and experimental work suggests that an interval. of at least six weeks should elapse between the extractions and radiation if the risk is to be reduced. It was hoped that the introduction of megavoltage radiotherapy would improve the situation but this has not been so if, as the higher dosages used still cause damage to bone. Six weeks is obviously too long to delay treatment for a malignant tumour and today opinions are divided as to the procedures to be adopted before radiotherapy is started. Some believe that all the teeth should be extracted before treatment except where the prognosis of the patient is poor. Others remove only those teeth which have advanced caries or periodontal disease and have turned their attention to preventing the need for further extractions. The need for meticulous oral hygiene is of the greatest importance, especially immediately after radiotherapy when the mouth becomes inflamed and sore. At this stage it is essential to supervise the oral hygiene closely, for discomfort may cause the patient to neglect regular cleansing. Topical fluoride applications may help but where caries and periodontal disease occur, both should be treated conservatively as soon as possible to save the teeth. Patients should be seen at three-monthly intervals, certainly for the first year or so, till their susceptibility to dental disease can be assessed. The use of saliva substitutes has been suggested to aid lubrication of the tissues.

When a tooth must be extracted it is necessary to communicate first with the radiotherapist concerned who will explain the significance of the treatment given and the area of the jaws affected. The dental treatment plan may then be agreed jointly. This must always include prophylactic measures such as an antibiotic cover for extractions, which it is wise to continue until healing is complete (three weeks). As dentures may traumatise the mucosa and predispose to breakdown and infection it is often advised that these should not be worn, and certainly not before consultation with the radiologist concerned.

Radiotherapeutic methods. Radical treatment is given to the smaller lesion with a good blood supply and will only succeed if the very high dose necessary for cure is concentrated on the tumour while the normal tissues are spared as far as is possible. An irradium needle implant attempts to do this by placing the source of radiation in the tumour as in carcinoma of the tongue. The normal tissues are protected by designing a mould to push them as far out of the way as possible or by shielding them with gold or lead screens built into the appliance. External methods of radiation use two or more beams of X-rays, or gamma rays, crossing at the centre of the tumour. The radiotherapist, helped by his physicist, plans the treatment fields to give the tumour a very much higher dose than that given to the surrounding tissues. This type of treatment may last for 4–6 weeks and gives rise to a thick membranous reaction in the mucosa membranes. The patient must be closely supervised during and after treatment.

Radiation may be given palliatively to relieve the patient's symptoms for such life as he has left. This may be a single treatment but is more often a five- or ten-day course of X-ray therapy to about three-quarters of the dose necessary to destroy the growth completely. This is usually reserved for very large tumours with extensive bone destruction, or widespread lymph node involvement, and the dose is limited because the normal tissues would not recover were a full dose given.

Chemotherapy

Chemotherapy has been a major advance in the management of some malignant diseases. When first introduced, drugs were only used when other types of treatment had failed. Chemotherapy as the primary form of treatment for lymphomas and some leukaemias has markedly improved the long-term survival rates of patients.

Although radiotherapy and surgery can eliminate the primary tumour it is now appreciated that these have often metastasised although there is no clinical evidence of this disease. In an attempt to prevent secondary tumours developing from metastatic deposits adjuvant chemotherapy is used in those malignant diseases which have a high propensity of metastatic spread.

Many drugs are now available and are administered in combination in high doses intermittently. The following are the main groups of chemotherapeutic drugs. The *alkylating agents* (nitrogen mustard, cyclophosphamide) react with essential cell constituents and produce damage. *Anti-metabolites* include the folic acid antagonists (methotrexate), antipyrimidines (5-fluorouracil) and antipurines (b-mercaptopurine); they interfere with the synthesis of essential cell constituents. The *Vinca alkaloids* (vincristine, vinblastine interfere with cell division. *Antibiotics* (actinomycin D, bleomycin) interact with DNA. *Platinum compounds* (cis-platinum) bind to DNA. *Corticosteroids* are widely used in combination with the above drugs.

The major side effects of chemotherapy are nausea and vomiting, bone marrow suppression, alopecia and stomatitis. To reduce the severity of the last complication a high standard of oral hygiene must be maintained and ill-fitting dentures relined or replaced.

Further reading

Binney, W. H., Cawson, R.A., Hill, G. B. and Soper, A. E. (1972), *Oral Cancer in England and Wales*. HMSO, London.
Henk, J. M. and Langdon, J. D. (1985), *Natural History, Response to Treatment and Prognosis in Malignant Tumours of the Oral Cavity*. Edward Arnold, London.

Lucas, R. B. (1984), *The Pathology of Tumours of the Oral Tissue*, 4th edn. Churchill Livingstone, Edinburgh.

Moore, J. R. (1986), *Surgery of the Mouth and Jaws*. Blackwell Scientific Publications, Oxford.

Pindborg, J. J. (1980), *Oral Cancer and Precancer*. John Wright, Bristol.

Souhami, R. L. and Tobias, J. S., eds. (1987), *Cancer and its management*. Blackwell Scientific Publications, Oxford.

Wright, B. A., Wright, J. M. and Binnie, W. H. (1988), *Oral Cancer: Clinical and Pathological Considerations*. CRC Press, USA.

XVI Treatment of surgical conditions of the salivary glands

The diseases of the salivary glands that may be treated by surgery are cysts, salivary calculi, infections, and tumours.

The minor salivary glands

Cysts

These occur in the lips or cheeks and less often in the floor of the mouth. Trauma, especially cheek or lip biting, causes stenosis of the duct and damming back of saliva, which may accumulate to form one of two kinds of cyst.

Mucus extravasation cysts. In these the mucus ruptures through the duct and pools in the adjacent connective tissue. The cyst has no epithelial lining, being contained by flattened connective tissue.

Retention cysts. More rarely the mucus is still contained in the epithelium lining the duct which balloons to form an epithelial lined cyst.

Diagnosis. They present as painless, smooth, bluish swellings obviously containing fluid. At intervals they burst, discharging their contents, but if untreated heal and form again. In the sublingual glands they may grow to a considerable size and are called ranulae (Fig. 92).

Treatment. Mucus cysts are better excised, though this is a delicate operation. The incision is made by drawing a scalpel blade lightly over the swelling and through the mucosa for a short distance beyond the lesion on each side. The cyst is gently freed by blunt dissection and the gland concerned is also removed to prevent recurrence. Often other glands are seen in the wound, and these too should be removed lest their ducts become blocked by scar tissue and give rise to new cysts. The ranula is more difficult to treat by excision but may resolve with adequate marsupialisation. The roof of the lesion is excised and the defect packed with a Whitehead's varnish pack to allow epithelialisation from the base.

Tumours

The commonest tumours are the locally invasive pleomorphic adenoma, and the malignant adenoid cystic and mucoepidermoid carcinomata.

Diagnosis. The pleomorphic adenoma occurs most frequently, seventy per cent of which are found in the palate, the rest in the upper lip or buccal mucosa. It presents as a painless nodule of rubbery consistency which is not fixed to either the overlying mucosa or the deeper structures. In the palate it is usually found to one side of the midline near the junction of hard and soft palates. It may reach a considerable size.

Fig. 92 Ranula of floor of mouth.

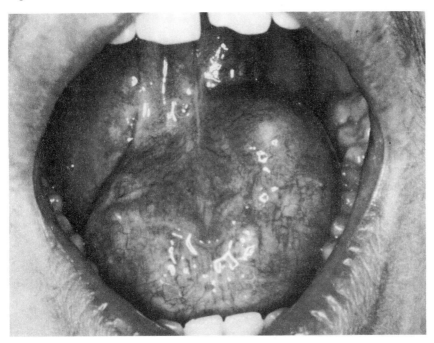

The adenoid cystic and mucoepidermoid carinomata resemble the pleomorphic adenoma clinically but may be of more rapid growth and show surface ulceration.

Treatment. The pleomorphic adenoma is treated by excision with a wide margin of normal tissue to remove tumour cells lying outside the capsule. Large defects may need skin or mucosal grafting. Adenoid cystic carcinoma may spread far along the perineural lymphatics so that treatment by excision has proved disappointing. Radiotherapy is often used because a larger volume of tissue can be treated without mutilation. Mucoepidermoid carcinoma is usually successfully treated by surgery or radiotherapy.

The major salivary glands

The diseases of the major salivary glands requiring surgery are obstructions to salivary flow, infections, and neoplasms.

Investigation of major salivary glands

Diagnosis. The chief complaints made by the patient are of pain, swelling, altered salivary flow and a bad taste. The periodicity and duration of the swelling is often of great assistance in making a diagnosis. The patient may express a subjective view of either an increase or decrease in salivary flow which it is difficult to confirm except by physiological methods of measurement which are not easy to perform.

Radiography. Radiographs in more than one plane are required. The submandibular gland is examined using a lateral oblique projection of the mandible with occlusal and posterior oblique views to show the duct. The parotid gland is seen on a postero-anterior film of the mandible with the central ray directed parallel to the ramus of the mandible, and on a lateral radiograph, taken with the head extended to avoid superimposition of the vertebral column. An orthopantomogram shows both glands.

In sialography a radiopaque contrast medium is used to show the network of ducts. By passing a fine cannula into the orifice of the duct the fluid is introduced under pressure equal to about 70-90 mm of water. This procedure must not be used where there is acute infection in the gland or until radiographs have excluded the presence of a stone. Sialographs reveal conditions not otherwise easily seen. Poorly calcified calculi show as filling defects, stenosis as narrowing of the duct, and tumours as an irregular filling pattern with areas of obliteration of the major and minor duct systems. The technique may be used with conventional radiographs and CT scans.

The use of scintiscanning has the advantage of examining all major salivary glands together. Following the intravenous injection of technetium the isotope is concentrated by the salivary glands. The head of the scanner picks up the radiation emissions and produces a picture of the glands.

Obstructions to salivary flow

Diagnosis

Obstruction to salivary flow may be caused by stenosis of the duct papilla, stricture of the duct, salivary calculi or pressure on the duct from a nearby lesion. The diagnostic symptom of obstruction is a recurrent painful swelling of the gland associated with meals or the sight of food. The swelling slowly goes down when the salivary stimulus is absent only to recur at the next meal. Calculi can often be directly palpated. The site and the nature of the lesion may be investigated by bimanual palpation, radiography, sialography and judicious probing using lacrimal dilators.

Treatment

Papillary stenosis more often affects the parotid papilla following trauma from dentures or the cusps of adjacent teeth. The submandibular duct may be affected where a salivary calculus causes chronic ulceration near the orifice. Treatment is by slitting the duct from its orifice for a short distance along its length and careful suturing of the margins to the surrounding mucosa.

Stricture remote from the papilla is not uncommon though the cause if unrelated to trauma is not always clear. The stricture may be dilated using a series of urethral bougies along the duct, but if this fails the stoppage is by-passed by surgery to bring the duct into the mouth proximal to the obstruction. Parotid strictures may require part of the duct to be reconstructed using a mucosal graft.

Fig. 93 Sialogram of submandibular salivary gland and duct.

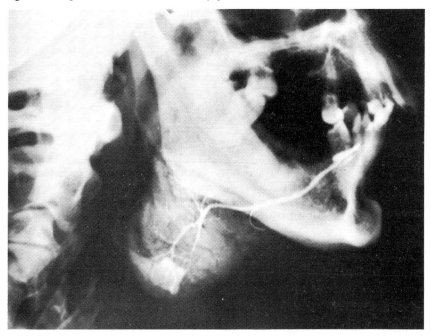

Sialolithiasis. The submandibular gland is affected three times more often than the parotid.

Submandibular calculi. The common sites for calculi are in the anterior two-thirds of the duct, in the posterior third at the distal border of the mylohyoid muscle and within the gland. Frequently they can be seen as a yellow swelling or felt on bimanual palpation inside and outside the mouth. Their presence should be confirmed by radiography.

Where an acute infection is present this should first be treated with antibiotics. Stones in the anterior two-thirds of the duct may be removed through an incision on the floor of the mouth. First the stone is accurately localised, by palpation, if possible. A suture is then passed deep to the duct and posterior to the stone. This is tied fairly tight to prevent the sialolith being pushed back into the gland. In operations on Wharton's duct an assistant should push up the floor of the mouth from below to improve access. An incision is made parallel to the duct which is found by blunt dissection and the calculus identified. The duct is incised and the stone removed. A fine catheter is then introduced into the lumen to aspirate any small remaining calculi. A free flow of saliva should be obtained, but as the duct may be stenosed anterior to the stone, a false opening is required where the incision was made. Small incision are left open, large ones are partially closed and where necessary a drain is used to create a new orifice. The patient is instructed to suck an acid drop every hour for a week to stimulate a flow of saliva from the gland to keep the new opening patent.

Stones in the posterior part of the duct may similarly be removed through an intraoral approach but this is a more difficult procedure needing a general anaesthetic and careful dissection to avoid damage to the lingual nerve which crosses the duct in this region.

Stones in the gland which cause symptoms are best treated by excising the gland.

Parotid calculi. These may occur anywhere in the duct or gland but as they are often poorly calcified they are not easily seen on plain radiographs. Calculi in the duct can be removed through an intraoral approach, but the course of the duct through the buccinator muscle makes the operation difficult. Stones lodged in the gland present particular problems. Those that give rise to only minor symptoms are best left untreated. Others may have to be removed by excision of the part of the parotid gland in which they lie.

Destruction of calculi at other sites in the body (e.g. renal) by ultrasound is now routine practice. As yet this technique (lithotripsy) has not been used on salivary calculi.

Fig. 94 *Above:* Radiograph of salivary calculus in submandibular salivary gland duct. *Below:* Calculus after removal.

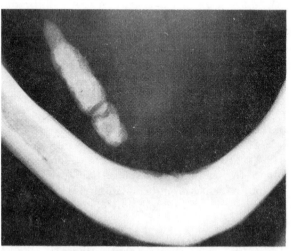

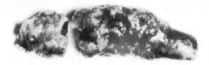

Sialadenitis

Acute sialadenitis

The parotid is more commonly affected than the submandibular gland and the sublingual rarely. Infection reaches the parotid gland through the duct and the predisposing factors are xerostomia, debilitation or disturbed function following abdominal surgery. The causal organism is usually staphylococcus.

Acute submandibular sialadenitis is almost invariably associated with a salivary calculus, or stricture of the duct.

Diagnosis. In acute infection the gland is swollen, tender or painful and the patient is febrile. In the submandibular gland pus may be seen discharging from the duct and the floor of the mouth on the affected side is red and swollen. The parotid gland rarely discharges pus through the duct though the papilla is often inflamed. The possibility of mumps should be considered.

Treatment. Severe gland infections should be admitted to hospital. Initially vigorous antibiotic therapy is instituted and where indicated incision and drainage performed. Salivary fistula rarely follows this procedure providing the skin incision is made a little away from the site of entry into the gland. Oral hygiene should be carefully supervised. Where no obvious cause is found a prolonged course of an antibacterial drug may be prescribed.

Chronic sialadenitis

Chronic infection frequently follows an acute attack, but may also result from prolonged obstruction to salivary flow. In the parotid this may be accompanied by sialectasis seen on sialography as dilatations of the ducts. Treatment consists of removing any suspected underlying cause, dilatation of strictures to encourage salivary flow using lacrimal dilators and antibiotic therapy. Where these fail excision of the submandibular gland is advised but excision of the parotid is deferred whenever possible because of the danger to the facial nerve.

Tumours

Of all the major salivary glands the parotid is most often the site of tumours, the commonest of which is the pleomorphic adenoma. This occurs ten times more often in the parotid than in the submandibular gland.

Diagnosis. The pleomorphic adenoma presents as a slowly enlarging, painless swelling. Sialography in the area shows obliteration of the normal duct structure. Malignant tumours present in the same way though later they may have additional symptoms of pain and, where the growth involves the facial nerve, a facial weakness according to the branch affected. Benign tumours in salivary glands are very rare.

Treatment. In view of the difficulty of differential diagnosis and the pre-dominance of the locally invasive and malignant tumours a biopsy is contraindicated as it may lead to spread of the disease. The treatment of choice in the parotid is to excise the tumour with a wide margin of normal tissue, or in the submandibular gland to excise the whole gland.

Excision of the submandibular gland. A curved incision about 7.5 cm long is made in a crease of the neck about 2.5 cm below the lower border of the mandible to avoid the mandibular branch of the facial nerve.

The underlying fascia and platysma are divided and the facial vessels found and ligated. With blunt dissection or using a finger the gland is separated from the connective tissue. In long-standing chronic cases this may be difficult due to fibrosis. The facial artery has to be ligated again on the posterior aspect of the gland. Superiorly the lingual nerve, which may be embedded in the capsule, gives off two small branches to the gland which are cut to free the nerve. The duct is dissected out, ligated as near the mouth as possible and cut, care being taken not to damage the lingual nerve. If excision is being done to remove a stone its presence on the excised gland should be confirmed before closure as it may easily slip out of the duct to be left in the wound. A vacuum drain is inserted prior to closure to reduce post-operative swelling.

Surgery of the parotid gland. The approach to this gland is made through a preauricular incision extending from the temporal region to the angle of the mandible. A facial flap is taken forward to expose the gland. The difficulty in excising the whole or part of the parotid is the facial nerve which runs in the substance of the gland and which if mishandled may leave the patient with a facial weakness or paralysis. During the dissection the auriculotemporal nerve may be damaged causing Frey's Syndrome, a profuse and embarrassing facial sweating which the patient suffers whenever he salivates.

Further reading

Anderson, R. and Byers, L. T. (1965), *Surgery of the Parotid Gland.* C. V. Mosby, St Louis.

Cohen, B. and Kramer, I. R. H., eds. (1976), *Scientific Foundations of Dentistry*, Ch. 44. Heinemann, London.

Mason, D. U. and Chisholm, D. (1975), *Salivary Glands in Health and Disease.* W. T. Saunders, London.

XVII The temporomandibular joint

Surgery of the temporomandibular joint is seldom the treatment of choice. Disorders of the joint have a multifactorial aetiology and successful management lies in careful assessment of the joint, the muscles moving the mandible and the relationship between the mandible and the maxilla. Treatment involves co-operation between restorative dentists, orthodontists and oral surgeons. Only when conservative treatments have been extensively tried but have failed is surgery considered.

It is useful to consider the frequency with which disorders of the joint present as this emphasises the nature of the clinical problem. The commonest conditions are acute trauma including dislocation, osteoarthrosis (a degenerative condition), pain dysfunction syndrome and structural internal derangement. Less common are systemic diseases involving the joint, principally rheumatoid arthritis, but polyarthritic psoriasis and ankylosing spondylitis do sometimes involve the joint, though it is uncommon for local symptoms to be the patient's chief complaint or the reason for seeking treatment. Rarely, developmental abnormalities such as agenesis or hyperplasia of the condyle, suppurative infections and tumours occur.

Diagnosis

This is made from the history, a careful examination of the joint, the muscles of mastication and of the occlusion, together with radiographs.

History. The history in acute trauma, dislocation and developmental abnormalities will strongly suggest the diagnosis. Internal derangement may result from trauma but this may be so insignificant (yawn or shout) that the patient is unaware of the event. Anterior displacement of the disc results in clicking and locking of the affected joint. By manipulation of the mandible, the patient can attain normal opening but with repeated trauma the disc becomes further displaced and the patient presents complaining of persistent restricted opening. Pain due to secondary muscle spasm occurs late in the progress of the disorder.

Where there is an increased load on the joint due to bruxism or a deficient occlusion the pain dysfunction syndrome may result. The patient complains of a click, pain and trismus. The click may resolve as the condition progresses as jaw opening is limited by muscle pain. Resolution of symptoms occurs when the increased loading (e.g. bruxism) ceases but returns if causative factors reappear. The pain dysfunction syndrome is now recognised as a cause for headaches. The syndrome occurs in patients of 15–30 years of age and females present for treatment more commonly than males, although symptoms are found to be present equally in both sexes.

Should an increased load on the joint persist, degenerative changes may occur, resulting in osteoarthrosis, usually seen in patients over 40 years of age. The symptoms are pain and trismus worsening with the use of the jaw as the day progresses. Pain is limited to the area of the joint and crepitus is always present. Acute symptoms indicate erosion of the condyle or bony fossa while during repair and remodelling the patient has little discomfort or trismus though the crepitus persists.

Examination. The joint is examined by palpating the condyles just anterior to the tragus where its movements can be felt. Placing the little finger into the external auditory meatus allows palpation of the posterior aspect of the joint. The range of condylar movement is compared to the excursions of the mandible in opening and lateral movements. Tenderness to pressure is noted both over the condyle head and posterior to it when the mouth is open. Clicking and crepitus are important and are more easily heard with a stethoscope. The masseter muscle is palpated in the cheek while the body of temporalis is examined, with teeth clenched, in the temple region. Palpation along the anterior border of the ascending ramus towards the coronoid process may elicit tenderness in the temporalis tendon. Opening or lateral movement against pressure from the surgeon's hand produces pain in the lateral pterygoid muscle. Typically the masseter is painful in those who clench whilst temporalis is painful in bruxists.

The range of opening of the mouth and lateral movements performed should be measured for comparison of later progress. The minimal, normal opening is considered to be 35 mm in females, 40 mm in males. Measurement may be undertaken with a Willis or Vernier bite gauge. Lateral movements are measured by comparing the mandibular centre line with the maxilla and if less than 8 mm, regarded as restricted. The teeth and occlusion are carefully charted and dentures assessed. Particularly important is whether centric relation and centric occlusion coincide. Any slide of the mandible from centric relation to centric occlusion and cuspal interferences on premolar or molar teeth are noted. Patient's occlusal habits such as clenching, protrusive movements or signs of bruxism such as attrition of the teeth, fractured cusps, ridging of the cheeks or scalloping of tongue are important.

Radiography. Satisfactory radiographs of the temporomandibular joint are difficult to take. Various views are used of which the transpharyngeal probably gives the best view of the condyle head. Interpretation also requires much experience as early changes are not easily identified or interpreted. Arthrography, where radio-opaque medium is injected into the joint space, gives an outline of the disc and shows displacement or perforation. Computerised tomography and magnetic resonance imaging techniques may aid diagnosis but in the commonest condition seen, the pain dysfunction syndrome, no changes are found by any imaging techniques.

Pain dysfunction syndrome

Clicking together with pain and limitation of movement constitute the temporomandibular joint pain dysfunction syndrome. It is associated with increased loading on the joint due to bruxism, clenching or occlusal interference. The onset of pain and trismus in many patients is related to muscle tenderness. Episodes of excessive bruxism and clenching, thought to be an emotional response, will lead to muscular pain. Clicking may be present only in the early stage of the syndrome and alone does not require treatment unless it causes the patient distress.

Treatment. Very many treatments have been advocated and much controversy still exists between supporters of the various schemes. Described here is a plan which has been advocated and known to be successful in treating the majority of patients suffering from the disorder. Counselling is important to explain the aetology and pathology of the condition and may help the patient to stop a daytime habit of clenching or bruxing. Resting the jaw by a soft diet and the use of anti-inflammatory drugs (Ibuprofen) will reduce pain. Care must be taken when prescribing these drugs to ensure that the patient has no medical history which contraindicates their use. Where doubt exists the advice of their general medical practitioner should be sought. Occasionally the symptoms are very acute when rest and the use of anti-inflammatory drugs are indicated. A splint may aid muscle relaxation.

Where the symptoms are more chronic, exercises to improve the pathway of opening may help the patient and prevent recurrence of the symptoms. To stop bruxism at night an occlusal interference splint placed on the teeth may break the habit. (Fig. 95). 25 mg Diazepam may be prescribed before retiring. Occlusal interference should be eliminated by a stabilisation splint which provides balanced contact between opposing teeth and, in eccentric movements (lateral and protrusive), takes the posterior teeth out of occlusion. Both these splints are worn at night for periods of 6–16 weeks, the patient weaning themselves off their use once they are symptom-free, after which consideration may be given to occlusal adjustments to the teeth by careful selective grinding or provision of prostheses. For these the patient is referred to a specialist in restorative dentistry.

Where occlusal treatments are unsuccessful, consideration should be given to the possibility that the pain may be psychological in origin and require more specific management such as specialist help and anti-depressant drugs. The patient's general medical practitioner should be consulted and asked to assist in treatment.

Osteoarthrosis

This is a degenerative condition of the articulating surfaces of the joint. Whereas in an inflammatory lesion the pathological process starts in the synovium and thence affects the bone, current evidence suggests that in osteoarthroses the primary disorder affects the subcondylar bone which becomes harder than normal, in turn affecting the overlying cartilage

Fig. 95 *Top*, occlusal interference splint. *Lower*, anterior repositioning splint.

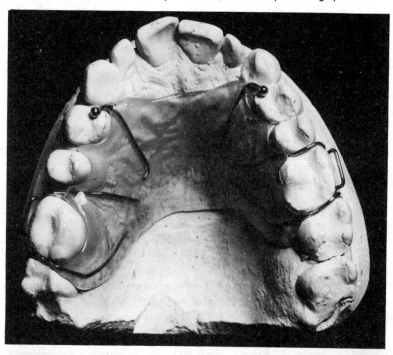

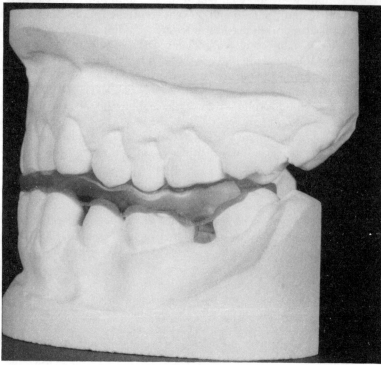

causing splitting, lipping and osteophytes. The disorder affecting the temperomandibular joint is probably secondary to trauma caused by overloading because of occlusal defects or bruxism. Epidemiological studies have shown degenerative lesions to be widespread among normal populations but patients only present for treatment when they experience pain possibly from a transient inflammatory episode.

Diagnosis. The symptoms are similar to those of the pain dysfunction syndrome, but the patients are usually over 40 years of age. The damaged joint surface produces a crunching sound (crepitus) on movement which can best be heard with a stethoscope. Erosions, when present, can sometimes be detected radiographically on the anterosuperior part of the condyle and its antagonistic area on the articular eminence.

Treatment. This is directed to relieving symptoms and prevention of further degeneration. Short-wave diathermy to the joint area and prescription of nonsteroidal anti-inflammatory drugs helps the pain and trismus. Reduction of the load on the joint by occlusal rehabilitation should help to prevent the disease progressing. When the pathological changes are advanced surgery may be indicated to remove the diseased condylar bone.

Internal derangement

Diagnosis is difficult from the history as this may be similar to that of the dysfunction syndrome. A history of trauma may be present but it may be so minor that the patient does not recollect the incident. Where the symptom of trismus fails to settle after the treatment described above displacement of the disc must be considered. The commonest derangement within the joint is anterior displacement of the disc, which impedes the movement of the condyle resulting in limited opening. Should opening and closing the mouth with the mandible protruded eliminate the click the diagnosis of a displaced disc is probable. The use of an anterior repositioning splint to aid diagnosis is then indicated.

Treatment. An anterior repositioning splint which holds the mandible-forward eliminates the symptoms (Fig. 95). To be effective the splint is worn all day and night and removed only for cleaning. After 8–10 weeks the splint is adjusted to result in the mandible being allowed to return to its usual position.

Occasionally, when the disc has been displaced for some time, treatment with a splint is unsuccessful and surgery to reposition the disc is indicated.

Dislocation of the condyle

Dislocation of the condyle occurs usually in a forward direction over the eminentia articularis, and is often bilateral. The predisposing cause is laxness of the capsule and associated ligaments of the joint which allows excessive movement when opening the mouth wide as in yawning. Normal joints may be dislocated by a blow particularly while the mouth is open. Under a general anaesthetic dislocation can be caused by opening the mouth with a gag, or by downward pressure when extracting lower teeth, if the support to the jaw is inadequate.

Diagnosis.   The patient complains of inability to bring the teeth together. In unilateral dislocation the midline of the mandible is deviated to the unaffected side. The dislocated condyle can be palpated in front of the eminentia articularis and radiographs confirm this position.

Treatment.   If reduction is attempted immediately it can usually be achieved without sedation or a general anaesthetic. However, if some time has elapsed muscle spasm may make reduction difficult and relaxation of the muscles will be necessary either by the use of intravenous diazepam or a general anaesthetic. The operator places his thumbs (protected from the teeth by binding with gauze) over the external oblique line or retromolar fossa of the mandible on each side. The remaining fingers are cupped under the chin. While the thumbs press down, the fingers lift up the chin to slip the condyle head back over the eminentia.

Chronic recurrent dislocation.   Where the capsule is very slack the condyle may dislocate several times a day. Many affected patients can reduce their mandibles at will, but others require it to be done for them. Surgery can be used for these chronic cases to restrict movement either by removing the eminetia, grafting bone over the eminetia to act as a stop, or by capsulorrhaphy, that is inserting fascial grafts or making a tuck in the capsule so that it is less lax. Alternatively the condyle head is excised.

Fractures of the condyle.   These are discussed in Chapter XIV.

Trismus

This is inability to open the mouth normally and with pain and clicking is one of the commonest symptoms associated with the temporomandibular joint and may be found in any of the conditions from which it suffers. As it is a symptom its cause should always be carefully sought, diagnosed and treated.

Persistent trismus may occur due to intra-articular fibrosis or bony ankylosis following trauma, infection or certain diseases such as rheumatoid arthritis. It may also be secondary to extra-articular fibrosis or scarring.

Intra-articular bony or fibrous ankylosis must be treated by surgery, either removal of the condyle (condylectomy) or cutting through the neck of the condyle (condylotomy). Trismus due to rheumatoid arthritis, ankylosing spondylitis or to extra-articular scarring may benefit from treatment with mechanical exercisers. In milder cases the patient can use an acrylic screw (Fig. 96) turned slowly to force the jaws apart. Alternatively, wooden spatulae in increasing numbers may be inserted between the teeth each day. In more severe conditions the jaws are prised apart with Mason's gags used bilaterally under a general anaesthetic. Impressions are taken and a prop placed between the teeth until an exerciser can be fitted. Once a satisfactory opening (2.5 cm measured between the incisor teeth) has been obtained, this is maintained by using an acrylic screw or wooden spatulae for about ten minutes each day for six months.

Fig. 96 *Top*, Trismus screw. *Lower*, shows screw in use.

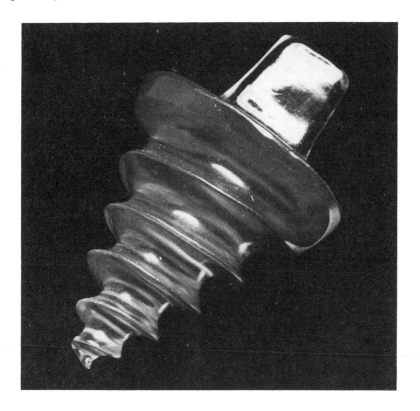

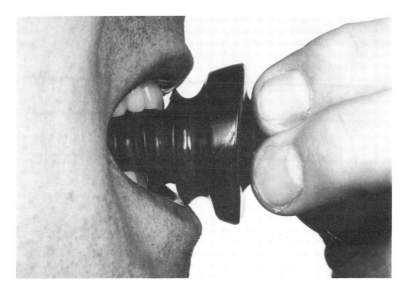

Surgery

Surgical procedures are undertaken rarely and only when conservative methods have failed. For osteoarthrosis with erosion of the condylar head *intracapsular condylectomy* removes the diseased bone. The new articulating surface becomes covered by fibrous tissue.

For internal derangement, *meniscal reattachment*, whereby the displaced disc is freed and reattached posteriorly, is performed. *Videoarthroscopy*, where adhesions are surgically cut, is finding a place in treatment.

Access to the joint

The joint cavity is limited above by the zygomatic arch and posteriorly by the external auditory meatus. Surgery is made difficult by the facial nerve which passes through the parotid gland (in which it is quite deeply buried) about 2 cm below the zygomatic arch, and by the internal maxillary artery deep to the joint. The condyle is accessible only through an area about 2 cm^2 and may be approached by a pre-auricular incision made in front of the tragus and above the attachment of the lobe of the ear up to the zygomatic arch and then obliquely up and forward for 2 cm, or by a post-auricular incision behind the ear which is then drawn forward to expose the joint (Fig. 97). The transverse facial and superficial temporal arteries may require ligation. The superior part of the parotid gland is drawn down, and the zygomatic arch cleared of the masseter. All stretching of the tissues to gain access is avoided lest it cause a facial nerve weakness.

Fig. 97 Surgical approach to the temporomandibular joint. Note *A*, facial nerve, *B*, superficial temporal artery, *C*, line of pre-auricular incision, *D*, line of pre-auricular incision through the tragus.

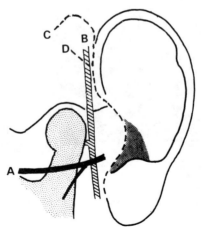

Further reading

Keith, D. A., ed. (1987), *Surgery of the Temporomandibular Joint.* Blackwell Scientific Publications, London.

Laskin, D. M. (1969), 'Aetiology of the pain dysfunction syndrome', *J. Am. Dent. Assoc.,* **79**, 147.

Ogus, H. D. and Toller, P. A. (1986), *Common Disorders of the Temporomandibular Joint,* 2nd edn. John Wright, Bristol.

Solberg, W. K. (1986), *Temporomandibular Disorders.* British Dental Journal publication.

xviii Occlusal and facial disharmony

Facial deformities may be congenital in origin, when they are usually bilateral, or they may be acquired as a result of trauma, infection, or radiotherapy. These may cause severe deformity if they occur during the period of development and involve the growth centres. In later life trauma and extensive surgery for malignant neoplastic disease are the commonest causes of bone destruction. The treatment of facial deformities is the province of the oral and maxillofacial surgeon and the plastic surgeon. In certain patients such as those with cleft palates the oral surgeon, orthodontist and plastic surgeon will work in close collaboration, in others the oral surgeon works with the orthodontist.

It is difficult to define a harmonious face as this varies from race to race and at different periods of time. However, today, gross disproportion of maxilla or mandible is regarded as ugly. An unacceptable appearance often goes with a poor occlusal relationship, Angle's Class I occlusion is associated with facial harmony while a gross Class II or III malocclusion may be accompanied by an unsightly appearance. It is important to realise that a mild degree of facial disharmony can be pleasing, and the temptation to give patients a stereotyped facial appearance, lacking in character, must be resisted. Consideration of the soft tissues overlying the bones is important as facial appearance is the consequence of the position of both hard and soft tissues.

Classification of occlusal and facial disharmony

The relation of the teeth to one another either in the same or in the opposing arch may be abnormal. This may be due to the malposition of individual teeth or of groups of teeth within a dental arch. These alveolar abnormalities, when gross, may present as localised pre- or post-normal occlusions or as conditions such as cross bite or open bite.

They must be distinguished from disproportionate growth of the skeletal bone which causes not only malocclusion but also disharmony between the middle and lower thirds of the face. The more common of these are shown in Table 8. One or more may occur together; thus anterior open bite is frequently associated with prognathism; unilateral overgrowth at the mandibular condyle leads to deviation of the midline towards the normal side and an open bite on the affected side. Bilateral overgrowth may result in a symmetrical prognathism with or without an open bite. The appearance of a protrusive lower jaw is the result of disproportion between the mandible and the maxilla and may be due to a combined deformity of a small maxilla with a large mandible. Identification of the site of the deformity is important before treatment is planned.

Table 8 Classification of commoner facial deformities

Site	Deformity	Occlusion
Mandible	Retrusive (Micrognathia)	Postnormal Angle Class II. Increased overjet.
	Protrusive with normal midline (Prognathism)	Prenormal. Reverse incisor overjet Angle Class III.
	Protrusive with deviation of midline (Prognathism)	Reverse incisal overjet Angle Class III. Midline of lower incisors deviated to one side. Cross bite.
	Anterior open bite (Apertognathia)	Vertical spacing between incisors with no overbite.
	Posterior open bite	Vertical spacing between premolar and molar teeth.
Middle third of face	Retrusive maxilla	Prenormal Angle Class III. Decreased or reverse overjet.
	Protrusive maxilla	Postnormal Angle Class II. Increased overjet.
	Retrusion of whole middle third face	Prenormal Angle Class III. Decreased or reverse overjet.

Combinations of alveolar and skeletal abnormalities are also quite common and must be distinguished by careful study of the occlusion, radiographs of the skull and facial bones and photographs of the face. Finally the possibility of a systemic condition such as a pituitary disorder, gigantism or acromegaly, or a local tumour or hyperplasia must always be considered.

Diagnosis and assessment

History. Many patients with occlusal or facial disharmony will be referred for a specific problem the management of which will be part of planned orthodontic treatment. Others will present with symptoms such as difficulty in chewing due to poor occlusion, inability to wear a lower denture or those associated with temporomandibular joint disorder. A complaint about facial appearance is sometimes made by the patient but, though this is the reason many seek treatment, few, in fact, mention it. As some skeletal abnormalities are hereditary it is important to ask about disharmony in other members of the family.

Examination. The face is first examined but care is necessary in drawing conclusions from this for, as shown in Table 8, quite different skeletal deformities can be found with similar changes in jaw relationship. A full clinical and radiographical examination is made of the mouth and teeth, particular care being taken to note those which are carious, periodontally involved or unerupted. Accurate impressions of the dentition are taken, the occlusion registered and models mounted on an anatomical articulator.

The interdigitation of the teeth in the mounted casts must be checked against the patient's mouth to ensure that no error has occurred in the laboratory which could lead to serious mistakes in diagnosis and treatment planning.

From these models misplaced teeth and alveolar abnormalities can usually be assessed but cephalometric radiographs and photographs are needed to differentiate them from skeletal abnormalities.

Lateral cephalometric radiographs are used to study the relationship of the upper and lower jaws to the cranial base and to each other. It is outside

Fig. 98 Lateral cephalometric radiograph of patient with prognathic mandible. Line from mid point of sella turcica (S) to the nasion (N), and thence to the point of maximum concavity anteriorly on the labial surface of the maxilla above the incisors (A) and the maximum concavity on the labial surface of the mandible below the incisors (B). In Angle Class I SNA = 80.5°; SNB = 76.6°; SNA − SNB = 3.9°; this is raised in Class II and reduced in Class III.

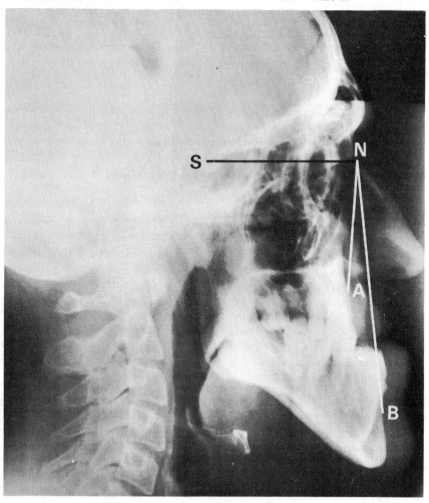

the scope of this book to give detailed cephalometric analysis. Fig. 98 gives a simple analysis using certain points on the bones to make measurements which aid diagnosis. Whilst the soft tissue outline can be seen on a cephalometric radiograph, more accurate information can be obtained from a transparency prepared from a photograph. This is taken with the head in a fixed position so that superimposition of photograph and radiograph may be achieved. Recent developments for assessment include the use of computer graphics to provide a three-dimensional picture of the face and head.

Lateral and full-face photographs not only are important in diagnosis and treatment planning but also provide a visible record of the effects of treatment.

Morphanalysis is another method by which photographs and radiographs can be superimposed and the relationship between the bones and soft tissue studied. Measurement of a large number of individuals has allowed a wide range of normal values to be developed for the head and face at different ages and these normal values can be used to identify the patients disharmony (Fig. 99).

Fig. 99 Superimposition of photographs and radiographs for morphanalysis.

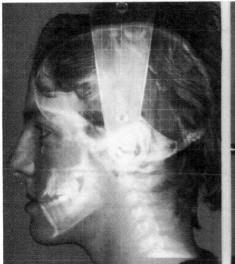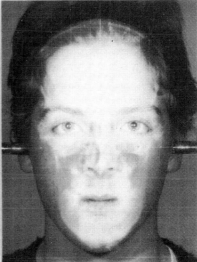

Treatment planning

The aim of treatment is to improve both the occlusion and the facial appearance. The final treatment plan may be a compromise between these to obtain a stable result which will not relapse. Before any surgical plan is made, orthodontic advice is sought to ensure that appliance therapy alone cannot give a satisfactory result. Further, for many patients orthodontic treatment before or after surgery is an integral part of treatment. All unerupted, carious, and periodontally involved teeth must be investigated and their treatment completed so that the true state of the occlusion is realised.

It is important that the patient fully understands what the operation entails, including possible complications, before they decide to proceed with treatment. Care must be taken to avoid guarantees for the results of the operation which are beyond the surgeon's power to deliver.

To enable the patient to appreciate what is involved they may be given the opportunity to meet a person who had has similar treatment to discuss their experience. This should be done in an informal atmosphere without the surgeon being present.

Alveolar surgery

Duplicate models of the patient's teeth can be sectioned to simulate the surgical procedures and examine their effect on the occlusion. Where bone cuts are to be made near structures such as the roots of the teeth or the mental foramen these, after careful study of the radiographs, may be drawn on the model (Fig. 100). The operation can then be designed to avoid damaging them.

Skeletal surgery

Planning is done by cutting photographs and radiographs to simulate possible surgical movements of the bones and consequent soft tissue positions. Accurate models of the mouth mounted on an anatomical articulator, cut at proposed surgical sites, are occluded in the new position to ensure that a satisfactory stable occlusion is obtained. Pre- or post-operative orthodontic treatment may be indicated to ensure a stable position which will not result

Fig. 100 Mandibular model marked up to show roots of teeth and mental foramen so that a bone cut, dashed line, is planned to avoid these strictures.

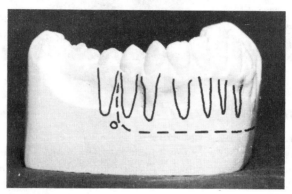

in post-operative relapse. In complicated deformities exact reproduction of the maxilla and mandible are made by registering the occlusion on a face bow with pointers at the midpoint of the chin and at the mandibular angles, Cephalometric radiographs are taken with the patient's teeth occluding on the bite of the face bow which carries radiopaque markers in the molar regions a set distance apart. From these films the dimensions of the mandible can be calculated and an accurate full-scale replica of the bone made in wax.

The patient can be shown the photographs of the expected post-operative result as an indication of the improvement which can be expected in their appearance. However, caution must be used when discussing this as it is difficult to be certain of the true post-operative soft tissue position.

Combined alveolar and skeletal surgery

In some patients a satisfactory result can be obtained only by combining skeletal surgery to the basal bones with alveolar surgery to move blocks of teeth.

Surgical procedures for the correction of deformities

Segmental surgery

In these procedures blocks of alveolar bone are separated surgically and repositioned. Where this takes place without removing bone it is known as an *osteotomy*, but where bony tissue has to be removed to achieve a satisfactory relationship, the term *osteotomy* is used. The blood supply to the separated portion including the pulps of the teeth is maintained by the soft tissues but the pulpal nerve supply is severed.

Segmental surgery combined with rapid orthodontic movement of the teeth or of blocks of bone and teeth is performed by making cuts through the cortical bone only *(corticotomy)*, the blood supply being maintained through the intact cancellous bone and the soft tissues. Rapid orthodontic movement of the segment by use of elastic bands or splints completes the procedure. The nerve supplying the pulps of the teeth is maintained in this operation.

Mandibular segmental osteotomy and osteotomy. The lower incisor teeth may be repositioned forwards by osteotomy or interiorly by osteotomy. A buccal mucoperiosteal flap is cut to expose the alveolus in the incisor and canine region. A vertical bone cut is made between the canine and premolar on each side and horizontally below the apices of the roots is removed beneath the apices of the roots. The bone is then repositioned and held by orthodontic bands and an arch wire or splints. The blood supply to the separated fragment is maintained by the lingual soft tissues.

Maxillary segmental osteotomy and ostectomy. A single tooth or teeth may be moved surgically in the maxilla. The commonest procedure is a push back operation of the six anterior teeth for maxillary protrusion.

The upper first premolar teeth are extracted. Buccal incisions are made in the mucoperiosteum and the maxillary bone is exposed along a narrow line from the lateral aspect of the floor of the nose, above the canine roots and down into the premolar sockets. A mucoperiosteal tunnel is also raised across the palate between the two first premolar sockets. A bone cut is made from the lateral aspect of the nose above the canine and down into the premolar socket. Palatal bone is removed across the palate between the two premolar sockets. The amount is determined from templates prepared pre-operatively on models. A small incision is made in the buccal sulcus between the upper central incisor teeth, the base of the nasal septum is identified and split off from the floor of the nose with a chisel. The piece of bone with the upper six front teeth is now freely mobile but retains its blood supply from the anterior buccal and palatal mucoperiosteum. The protrusive premaxilla is retropositioned and fixed by means of locking plates attached to splints on the anterior and posterior teeth or using orthodontic bands and an arch wire (Fig. 101).

Fig. 101 *Left:* Model of patient with maxillary protrusion, showing tooth to be extracted (hatched) and proposed line of bone section and bone to be removed (black) to allow anterior part of maxilla to be set back. *Right:* Planned result after repositioning.

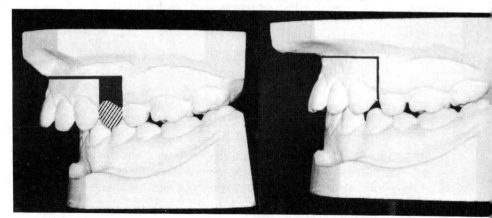

Skeletal surgery

Operations may be on the mandible or middle third of the face, and for some patients on both jaws, when it is termed *bimaxillary* surgery.

Mandibular prognathism. Many procedures have been devised for retropositioning the mandible but only those commonly used today will be described. These are operations on the ascending ramus and on the mandibular body. The decision to operate in the ramus or on the body is made from a study of the occlusion. Where a normal relationship exists between the mandibular and maxillary posterior teeth, but there is a reverse incisor bite, the anterior part of the mandible only need be retropositioned. This is done by removing a section of the body (ostectomy) on each side and setting the anterior part back. For the operation accurate templates must be prepared from models to indicate the extent and shape of the piece of bone to be removed. The teeth in the line of section are extracted and the operation performed via an intraoral approach. Alveolar bone is removed down to the inferior dental canal. The lower border of the mandible is identified and bone removed from below the inferior dental canal. The neurovascular bundle is carefully preserved and a small recess prepared to receive it. The bone ends are held in apposition with intraosseous wires and intermaxillary fixation (Fig. 102).

Fig. 102 *Mandibular osteotomies:* (a) and (b) subsigmoid osteotomy showing line of cut and overlapping of posterior fragment after retropositioning the mandible; (c) Saggital splitting of lower part of ascending ramus with removal of part of the buccal outer plate at A. This provides a large are of bone apposition after the lingual fragment has been slid back (Obwegeser). (d) Osteotomy of body to alow reposition of anterior part. Note small box cut in bone to accommodate the inferior dental nerve which is present.

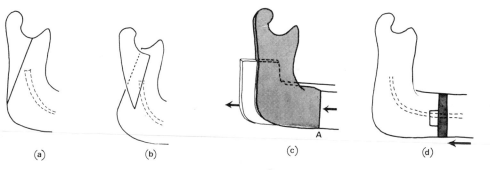

The majority of operations for the correction of prognathic mandible are based in division of the ascending ramus. This is exposed either intraorally through an incision over the anterior aspect of the ramus or extraorally, the incision being placed 2.5 cm below the angle of the mandible. The most popular procedures today for repositioning the mandible are the subsigmoid osteotomy and the sagittal split osteotomy (Obwegeser's operation).

For the subsigmoid osteotomy the ramus is divided from the sigmoid notch downwards and backwards behind the lingula to the posterior border at the angle of the mandible. The posterior fragment is brought laterally so that it lies outside the anterior portion which has been moved backwards (Fig. 99). This is most important for, if the posterior fragment lies inside the anterior, it will be displaced medically by the pull of the lateral pterygoid muscle and non-union with relapse or development of an anterior open bite can occur after the fixation is removed. Intraosseous wires are not generally necessary after this procedure but the mandible is immobilised by intermaxillary fixation.

The sagittal spilt osteotomy is employed where a large area of bone contact is required after retropositioning of the mandible. This is performed by an intraoral route and a vertical bone cut is made through the buccal cortical bone in the molar region and horizonally through the lingual cortical plate above the lingue on the ramus a sagittal cut is then made along the anterior border of the ascending ramus and, with an osteotome, the ramus is split sagitally. The body of the mandible and lingual portion of the ramus are retropositioned and a piece of buccal bone removed from the outer fragment so that it fits against the lingual portion. Intraosseous wires are passed and intermaxillary fixation applied (Fig. 102).

Anterior open bite. This occurs with other deformities particularly mandible prognathism and may be corrected at the same procedure as the retropositioning of the mandible. Where only an anterior open bite is present or it is accompanied by a mild prognathism, surgery of the mandibular body is indicated. This can be done by a cut made between the premolar teeth and then obliquely downwards and forwards below the apices of the teeth. The alveolar fragment is moved upwards and a bone graft inserted beneath it. This can be taken from the chin if it is prominent and needs reduction.

Mandibular retrusion. The majority of these cases are mild and do not require surgery, When severe the mandible may be lengthened by the sagittal split operation as described for mandibular prognathism, the mandible being drawn forwards, and no bone is removed from the buccal side of the distal outer fragment.

Where the dental occlusion is satisfactory but the chin is retrusive this can be improved by a bone graft.

Retrusive maxilla and middle third of the face. Surgically the facial bones can be sectioned at the Le Fort I, II, and III levels.

The Le Fort I osteotomy allows a retrusive maxilla to be brought forward and can also be used to treat an anterior open bite. Incisions are made bilaterally through mucoperiosteum to expose the maxillary bone above the apices of the teeth. A bone cut is made from the anterior nares to the tuberosity. The nasal septum and the lateral wall of the nose are divided with as osteome. This leaves the maxilla attached only to the ptergoid plates from which it can be gently freed using a curved osteotome. The maxilla is grasped in forceps and drawn forward. Bone grafts are inserted between the maxillary tuberosity and the pterygoid plates. The jaw is immobilised as described for a fractured maxilla.

The Le Fort II osteotomy allows the central part of the face to be brought forward. Incisions are made through skin and periosteum bilateraely in the medial canthal region and intraorally in the upper buccal sulcus. A bone cut is made from just below the frontonasal suture, across the lacrimal bone to the infraorbital ridge and downwards and posteriorly across the maxilla to the tuberosity, care being taken not to damage the infraorbital nerve and the lacrimal gland and duct. The two cuts are joined across the bridge of the nose. With a chisel, the bone is freed from the pterygoid plates and brought forward and immobilised as described for a fractured maxilla.

Patients with complex deformities involving the central part of the face, malar bones and orbits require a Le Fort III osteotomy.

Bone grafts

Where trauma or disease have caused loss of mandibular bone this may be replaced by a bone graft. The most satisfactory are of autogenous bone taken from the iliac crest or from the ribs. The iliac crest is more commonly used in this country as it provides a large area of medullary bone which can be cut to a satisfactory shape to fill most deformities. Homogenous grafts, taken from a person other than the patient, specially prepared and stored frozen, have also been used successfully. Sliding or pedicle bone grafts have been advocated. These are cut from the lower border of the mandible and, with their periosteum still attached, are slid across to make up the defect. Infection, gross contamination from the mouth and recent radiotherapy are direct contraindications to bone grafting.

Free grafts. Intermaxillary fixation is prepared, preferably using cast metal splints. The operation is best performed through an extraoral approach though the intraoral route has been successfully used.

In old deformities the mandible is exposed and the free ends identified. This may be difficult if they have displaced lingually into the soft tissues. The bone ends are stripped of periosteum and all scar tissue is excised.

The cortical plate is removed from the buccal or lingual aspect of the bone ends to form a step into which the iliac or rib graft, carefully trimmed to the right shape and size, is placed and fixed with interosseous wiring. The gap between the bone ends is then packed with cancellous chips. The wound is closed and the mandible kept immobilised for six weeks. Antibacterial drugs should be prescribed for a fortnight from the day of operation.

Microvasular surgery. A suitably shaped piece of cortical bone from the iliac crest accompanied by its blood vessels can be used to replace a missing portion of mandible. The blood vessels are anastamosed to the facial artery and vein, the surgery being done under a microscope. The graft thus acquires an immediate new blood supply.

Further reading

Henderson, D. (1985), *A Colour Atlas of Orthognathic Surgery*. Wolfe Medical Publications, London.

Moore, J. R. (1986), *Surgery of the Mouth and Jaws*. Blackwell Scientific Publications, Oxford.

Rabey, G. P. (1977), 'Current principles of morphanalysis and their implications in oral surgery practice', *Brit. J. Oral Surg.*, **15** , 97.

Appendix

Some normal haematological values: variation in health in adults

Red Cells
   Men: $4.5-6.5 \times 10^{12}/l$
   Women: $3.9-5.6 \times 10^{12}/l$

Haemoglobin
   Men: 13.5–18.0g/dl
   Women: 11.5–16.4g/dl

Mean corpuscular haemoglobin: 27–32 pg
Mean corpuscular haemoglobin concentration: 30–35g/dl
Packed cell volume
   Men: 0.40–0.54
   Women: 0.36–0.47

Leucocytes
   Adults: $4.0-11.0 \times 10^9/l$

Differential leucocyte count (adults)
   Neutrophils – 40–75%: $2.5-7.5 \times 10^9/l$
   Lymphocyte 30–45%: $1.5-3.5 \times 10^9/l$
   Monocytes 2–10%: $0.2-0.8 \times 10^9/l$
   Eosinophils 1–6%: $0.04-0.4 \times 10^9/l$
   Basophils less than 1%: $0.0-1.0 \times 10^9/l$

Platelets: $200-350 \times 10^9/l$

Some normal values in biochemistry

Sodium	132–144 mmol/l
Potassium	3.5–5.0 mmol/l
Bicarbonate	24–32 mmol/l
Calcium	2.10–2.70 mmol/l
Inorganic Phosphate	0.7–1.4 mmol/l
Albumin	38–48 g/l
Cholesterol	3.6–7.0 mmol/l
Protein (total)	50–80 g/l
Alkaline phosphatose	70–330 u/l
Blood glucose (fasting):	3.0–6.0 mmol/l
Blood urea:	2.5–7.5 mmol/l
(increases with age)	

Urine
    Specific gravity: 1.015–1.020
    Sugar: nil
    Protein: nil
    Ketones: nil

Cerebrospinal fluid
    Protein: 0.10–0.45 g/l
    Glucose: 2.0–4.5 mmol/l

Index

Abscess
  dental   144
  drainage of   68
  periapical   149
  subperiosteal   149
  treatment of   145
Acquired immune deficiency
  syndrome (AIDS)   30
Actinomycosis   159
Adenoid cystic carcinoma   221
Adrenal corticosteroids   20
Adverse drug reactions   48
Alveolar ridge augmentation   137
Alveolectomy   131, 133
Ameloblastoma   212
Anaemias   24
Anaesthesia
  choice of   60
  in acute infection   146
  in fractures   187
  in haemorrhagic disorders   28
Analgesics   44
Anaphylactic shock   33
Angioedema   22
Anterior open bite   244
Antibiotic agents   45
Anticoagulants   27
Apicectomy   164
Arch wiring   191
Artificial respiration   34
Asepsis   60
Aspiration   145, 163
Asthma   29

Barrel bandage   184
Biopsy   208
Blood
  anaemia   24
  anticoagulants   27
  clotting of   28
  haemorrhagic diseases   28
  leukaemia   25
  normal values   246
Bone
  cutting of   63
  generalised diseases of   30
  grafts of   245
  osteomyelitis   154
  substitutes   139

Bronchitis   29
Bruxism   227

Calcium hydroxyapatile   139
Calculi, salivary   223
Canines, maxillary unerupte   96, 108
Cardiac
  arrest   36
  failure   22
  massage   36
Cellutitis   144, 154
Cerebral vascular accidents   38
Chemotherapy   218
Chisels, use of   63
Computerised tomography   208
Condylar fractures   189
Conjunctivitis, post-operative   15
Consent to operative procedure   9, 10
Coronary heart disease   23
Corticosteroids   20
Craniomaxillary fixation   194
C.T. Scanning   208
Cysts
  aspiration   163
  assessment of   163
  classification of   160, 169
  diagnosis   160
  mucus   220
  radiography   161
  treatment of   164

Day-stay surgery   8, 16, 60
Death in the surgery   38
Debridement of wounds   68
Dental engine   49
Denture hyperplasia   137
Dentures, immediate   130
Dermoid cyst   170
Detached meniscus   234
Diabetes   21
Diagnosis   5, 6
Diet following oral surgery   10, 11, 12
Dislocation of T.M.J.   231
Drains   68
Dry socket   125

Elevators for extractions   80, 101
Emergencies in oral surgery
  anaphylactic shock   33

cardiac arrest   36
cerebral vascular accidents   38
coronary thrombosis   23
corticosteroid shock   20
diabetic coma, insulin shock   21
epileptic fits   30
fainting   32
fractures of jaws   183
haemorrhage   28
oroantral fistula   116
respiratory obstruction   34
surgical shock   33
Emphysema, surgical   125
Endocarditis   23
Enucleation of cysts   164
Epilepsy   30
Examination of the mouth   3
Eyelet wiring   190
Eyes   126

Facial disharmony
   classification   238
   diagnosis   239
   surgery   240
   treatment planning   239
Fainting   32
Fascial planes   151
Fever, post-operative   14
Fistula, oroantral   116
Fluid balance   10
Forceps, dental extraction   76
Fractured jaws
   anaesthesia for   187
   applied anatomy   172
   complications of
      delayed union   202
      infection   203
      malunion   203
      non-union   203
      residual trismus   204
   control of infection   183
   diagnosis   176, 178, 179
   emergency care   183
   immobilisation
      arch wiring   191
      barrel bandage   184
      circumferential wiring   200
      craniomaxillary fixation   194
      eyelet wiring   190
      intraosseous wiring   196
      plating   198

splints, Gunning's   200
splints, metal cap   192
transalveolar wiring   200
malar   189
mandible   172
   condyle   173
maxilla   174
radiography   178
reduction   187
repair of bone   185
soft tissue wounds   188
tuberosity   123
Fractured teeth   114
Fraenectomy   136

Giant cell reparative granuloma   211
Globulomaxillary cyst   170
Gowning up   54

Haemangioma   205, 212
Haemophilia   26
Haemorrhage
   arrest of   66, 91, 124
   clotting agents   92
   post-extraction   91, 124
Haemorrhagic diseases   25
Halo head frame   194
Head injuries   184
Hepatitis   29
History taking   1
Hospital in-patient care   56
Human Immune Deficiency
   syndrome   30
Hypertension   24
Hyperthyroidism   20

Immediate restoration dentures   130
Impacted teeth   93
Implants   140
Infections
   acute   145
      antibacterial drugs   146
      drainage   146, 68
      Ludwig's angina   154
      mandible   153
      maxilla   153
      maxillary in infants   157
      osteomyelitis   154
      periapical, dental   149, 158
      pericoronitis   148
      prevention   73
      salivary glands   225

spread through fascial
    planes 150
  subperiosteal abscess 149
  treatment, principles of 145
chronic 158
  actinomycosis 159
  periapical 158
  syphilis 159
  tuberculosis 158
Infective endocarditis 23
In-patient care 9
Instruments
  care of 50
  packs 52
  sterilising 51
Intensive care 16
Internal derangement T.M.J. 231
Interosseous fixation of fractures 196

Keratocyst 160

Laser surgery 210
Le Fort fractures 174
Leukaemia 25
Leukoplakia 206
Local anaesthesia with sedation 43
Ludwig's angina 154
Lymphadenitis 151
Lymph nodes 3, 151, 158

Magnetic resonance imaging
  (M.R.I.) 208
Malar fractures 189
Mandibular deformity
  protrusion 242
  retrusion 244
  treatment planning 239
Mandibular fractures 172
Marsupialisation 167
Maxillary retrusion 244
Maxillary sinus (antrum) 3
Menstruation 19
Microvascular surgery 215, 245
Micturition 12

Nasal antrostomy 120

Occlusal disharmony
  classification 238
  diagnosis 239
  surgery 241
  treatment planning 240

Oedema, post-operative 126
Open bite, anterior 244
Operating room and theatre 49
Oral hygiene 13
Oroantral fistula 116
Osseointegrated implants 141
Osteoarthrosis 228, 229
Osteomyelitis 154
Osteoradionecrosis 216
Osteotomy
  mandibular 243
  maxillary 244
Out-patient care 16

Packs for sockets 48
Paget's disease 30
Parotidectomy 226
Pericoronitis 148, 93, 99
Pharyngitis, post-operative 15
Platelets – disorders of 26
Plating – fractures 198
Pleomorphic adenoma 221, 225
Post-extraction haemorrhage 28
Post-operative
  care 17
  complications 14
  instructions 18
  out-patients 17
Pregnancy 19
Pre-operative care
  medication 42
  outpatients 17
Prognathism 239, 242
Prosthetic joints and valves 24
Prosthetic surgery
  alveolectomy 13
  deepening of the sulci 137
  dental irritation hyperplasia 137
  fraenectomy 136
  implants 140
  ridge augmentation 139
  torus palatinus 132
Pulmonary post-operative
  complications 15

Radiation – effects of 215
Radiotherapy 217
Ranula 220
Respiratory obstruction 34
Retractors 64
Rheumatoid arthritis of T.M.J. 228

Root in antrum 120
Roots, extraction of 88

Sagittal split osteotomy 243
Salivary glands
    calculi 223
    cysts 220
    infections of 225
    tumours 225
Scintisan 222
Scrubbing up 54
Sedation
    pre- and post-operative 42, 44
    with local anaesthesia 43
Septic socket 125
Sialoadenitis 225
Sialography 222
Sickle cell anaemia 24
Sleep 13
Special investigations 5, 7
Splints
    Gunning's 200
    metal cap 192
    T.M.J. disorders 231
Submandibular salivary glands
    diseases of 223
    removal 226
Suction apparatus 49
Sulcus, deepening of 137
Supernumerary teeth 91
Surgical sieve 5
Surgical shock 33
Surgical team 52
Suturing 70
Syphilis of jaws 159

Temporomandibular joint
    diagnosis 227
    dislocation 232, 123
    examination 228, 3
    meniscus 234
    osteoarthrosis 228
    pain dysfunction syndrome 229
Thalassaemia 25
Third molars unerupted 95, 102, 107
Tongue 4
Tonsils 4
Tooth extraction
    alveolectomy following 131, 133

assessment for extraction 75
complications of
    abnormal resistance 113
    dislocation of T.M.J. 123, 232
    emphysema, surgical 125
    extraction of wrong tooth 113
    fractured jaw 123
    fractured needle 127
    fractured teeth 88, 114
    fractured tuberosity 123
    haemorrhage 124
    infected tooth socket 124
    loss of tooth or roots 115
    oroantral fistula 116
    pain 126
    root in antrum 120
    soft tissue damage 122
    swelling 126
    trismus 126
deciduous teeth 79
elevators, dental 80, 101
forceps, dental 76
Torus palatinus 132
Tracheostomy 35, 147
Transalveolar approach 61, 88
Trismus 113, 126, 147, 232
Tuberculosis of jaws 158
Tuberosity, reduction of 135
Tumours
    benign, treatment of 211
    biopsy 208
    diagnosis 205
    locally invasive, treatment of 211
    malignant, treatment of 213
    of salivary glands 225

Unerupted teeth
    assessment 99
    radiography 95
    treatment 98
        canines, maxillary 109
        exposure 98
        extraction 99, 108
        mandibular third molars 102
        maxillary third molars 107
        supernumerary teeth 111

Vestibuloplasty 138
von Willebrand's disease 27
Vomiting, post-operative 14, 44

Acknowledgements

For this fourth edition we wish to thank the many clinicians and students past and present who have made useful comments and suggestions to improve the text, particularly Mr R. J. M. Gray of Manchester University for advice on the chapter on the temporamandibular joint. Chapters as indicated over the names in the contents list were written by Professor J. W. Frame of Birmingham University, Mr J. Cowpe of the University of Dundee and Mr U. J. Moore of Newcastle University. Nevertheless all errors and omissions remain our responsibility. We would like to express our gratitude for permission to use the following figures: Fig. 29 from Lomax, A. M. (1975), 'Extraction techniques for low seated dentistry', *Brit. Dent. J.* 138, 253. Fig. 96 from Dr G. P. Rabey, Department of Anatomy, University of Manchester. Figs. 80 & 85 from Mr J. E. Hawkesford, Newcastle General Hospital.

Several secretaries have been involved in producing the text: we wish to express our thanks to all of them.